# DEEPENING GROUP PSYCHOTHERAPY WITH MEN

# DEEPENING GROUP PSYCHOTHERAPY WITH MEN

## Stories and Insights for the Journey

FREDRIC E. RABINOWITZ

AMERICAN PSYCHOLOGICAL ASSOCIATION
Washington, DC

Published by
American Psychological Association
750 First Street, NE
Washington, DC 20002
www.apa.org

APA Order Department
P.O. Box 92984
Washington, DC 20090-2984
Phone: (800) 374-2721; Direct: (202) 336-5510
Fax: (202) 336-5502; TDD/TTY: (202) 336-6123
Online: http://www.apa.org/pubs/books
E-mail: order@apa.org

In the U.K., Europe, Africa, and the Middle East, copies may be ordered from
Eurospan Group
c/o Turpin Distribution
Pegasus Drive
Stratton Business Park
Biggleswade, Bedfordshire
SG18 8TQ United Kingdom
Phone: +44 (0) 1767 604972
Fax: +44 (0) 1767 601640
Online: https://www.eurospanbookstore.com/apa
E-mail: eurospan@turpin-distribution.com

Typeset in Meridien by Circle Graphics, Inc., Reisterstown, MD

Printer: Sheridan Books, Chelsea, MI
Cover Designer: Beth Schlenoff, Bethesda, MD

**Library of Congress Cataloging-in-Publication Data**
Names: Rabinowitz, Fredric Eldon, 1956- author.
Title: Deepening group psychotherapy with men : stories and insights for the journey / by Fredric E. Rabinowitz.
Description: Washington, DC : American Psychological Association, [2019] | Includes bibliographical references and index.
Identifiers: LCCN 2018047049 (print) | LCCN 2018047918 (ebook) | ISBN 9781433829451 (eBook) | ISBN 1433829452 (eBook) | ISBN 9781433829444 (hardcover) | ISBN 1433829444 (hardcover)
Subjects: LCSH: Group psychotherapy. | Men—Psychology. | Men—Mental health.
Classification: LCC RC488 (ebook) | LCC RC488 .R33 2019 (print) | DDC 616.89/15200811—dc23
LC record available at https://lccn.loc.gov/2018047049

**British Library Cataloguing-in-Publication Data**
A CIP record is available from the British Library.

*Printed in the United States of America*

http://dx.doi.org/10.1037/0000132-000

10 9 8 7 6 5 4 3 2 1

# CONTENTS

# FOREWORD

Sam V. Cochran

I invite you to join Dr. Fredric E. Rabinowitz on a journey into the inner workings of a men's therapy group. *Deepening Group Psychotherapy With Men,* by the psychotherapist who has written more than any other group therapist on working with men in groups, is a detailed application of the Deepening model of psychotherapy with men that he and I developed for individual psychotherapy. Deepening, as we use the term in therapy, is both an action verb characterizing the activity of the therapist during the therapy process and a description of how men are healed by discovering in some depth their hopes, fears, losses, frustrations, and traumas.

*Deepening Group Psychotherapy With Men* is a distinctive and invaluable contribution to the literature on psychotherapy with men in two important ways. First, it is the only book on group psychotherapy with men to weave together an explicit conceptual framework on working with men, the Deepening framework, with practical guidance for moment-to-moment and session-to-session interventions by the group therapist. Dr. Rabinowitz deftly illuminates the Deepening framework every step of the way and provides vignettes illustrating how the framework comes alive with the men in his therapy groups.

This book also provides an in-depth look into Dr. Rabinowitz's thoughts and observations over the life of a men's group. We glean his insights into the group members from their individual therapy experiences. We follow his thought process with regard to the selection of the group members. We join him as he provides an ongoing analysis of the unfolding group process over a 9-month course of weekly group meetings. Readers literally engage in the Deepening process by accompanying Dr. Rabinowitz as he unpacks the steps of group member selection and debriefs each group meeting with extensive commentary.

As the only book available to therapists that combines the conceptual foundation of the Deepening model with detailed session-to-session descriptions of the model as it plays out in a group of men, *Deepening Group Psychotherapy With Men* is a valuable and necessary book for therapists who are working with or who plan to work with men in the therapy group setting.

# ACKNOWLEDGMENTS

This book has been a labor of love. I have wanted to capture my experience as a group psychotherapist with men for a long time. With the blessing of the University of Redlands, where I have been employed as a professor since 1984, I was able to use my recent sabbatical year to write the first draft of this manuscript. It is important that I acknowledge Dr. Thomas Elliott, my best friend and coleader of the men's group for 30 years. His recent retirement has left me leading the group by myself, but his influence as my confidant over the years has enhanced my understanding of how to best work with men in this setting. My colleague and dear friend Dr. Sam Cochran has been my coauthor of much of my writing over the years. His insightful creativity and scholarship make up the theoretical underpinnings of the Deepening psychotherapy model that I have used in this book.

I am indebted to the men and women of Division 51, the Society for the Psychological Study of Men and Masculinities of the American Psychological Association. This organization has been a supportive home for me as I have interacted with clinicians, researchers, and students about the exciting field of male psychology.

The hundreds of men who have been a part of my individual practice and men's groups over the past 34 years are the inspiration for this book. Although I have disguised the identities of these amazing individuals, the characters I depict are based on my interactions with these courageous men. They have shown me their vulnerability, resilience, capacity for growth, and psychological depth.

I am in appreciation of my colleagues who reviewed the manuscript. They gave me excellent feedback that improved the readability, cohesiveness, and comprehensiveness of the book. I also thank my manuscript editor,

Susan Herman, for her detailed review and insight into how to best convey my ideas, and Amy Snyder, my copyeditor, for her careful read and detailed editing.

Finally, I am indebted to my family for their support on this project. My partner, Janet, gave me the space, time, and needed encouragement. My children, Karina and Jared, remind me of how important it is to document what I do so that another generation can gain some wisdom from this one. My mother, Barbara, continues to show me what lies ahead in this wonderful life journey.

# DEEPENING GROUP PSYCHOTHERAPY WITH MEN

# Introduction

## *Masculinities in Transition*

Gender roles for men and women worldwide have shifted dramatically in the last half century. Although men in power still hold privileged advantages in commerce, politics, and economic status, the tide has been turning toward gender equality. In the not-so-distant past of the mid-20th century, masculinity was defined by a fairly rigid code. This code included an expectation of male dominance and leadership in most aspects of life, a form of traditional masculinity buttressed by the predominantly patriarchal social forces. Men were assumed to be the primary providers and protectors of the family and community. Often they were oblivious to the power they wielded, especially with those who were not as privileged. Many men enacted these roles with little regard for unintended physical and psychological consequences (Kimmel, 2017). Historically, being a successful man in Western societies included self-reliance, strength, aggressiveness, and emotional stoicism in the face of pain, loss, and life challenges. Women were in charge of child care and the family, whereas men earned the money to provide and protect. Although problematic in countless ways, these gender roles also provided explicit structure for how to act as a man or woman.

### A DIFFICULT TRANSITION FOR MEN

The societal shifts that rocked traditional gender roles occurred relatively quickly in the late 1960s and 1970s. Many men, trained to be society's breadwinners, warriors, and protectors, were caught in the cultural undertow as

---

http://dx.doi.org/10.1037/0000132-001
*Deepening Group Psychotherapy With Men: Stories and Insights for the Journey,*
by F. E. Rabinowitz

women entered the workforce and demanded equal rights. Women struggled to break into a male-dominated labor market, but they did so with excitement, promise, and commitment to being included. Many men, on the other hand, were often on the defensive, displaced and confused by their less dominating new roles. To them, it felt as if something had been taken away. The patriarchal power they had taken for granted was being challenged. With women in the workforce, there was new competition for jobs and a new gendered dynamic in work relationships (Kimmel, 2017).

As the nature of work moved away from physical labor to a more technology-based foundation in the later part of the 20th century, education became more important than physical strength. In the current era, women attain degrees beyond high school in higher numbers than men (U.S. Department of Education, National Center for Education Statistics, 2017). Advanced education is now a requirement for many positions, and the shrinking physical labor market, requiring less education, is dependent on fluctuations in the health of the economy.

Although some men are (perhaps unknowingly) working hard to try to maintain the male-led social structure in which they feel most comfortable, the older model of masculine dominance is no longer being supported by society's values and economic engine. Unless men make the shift to a more flexible orientation in terms of control, power, and decision making at work and in relationships with women, they risk dangerous consequences such as crumbling relationships with their partners, high levels of psychological stress, and physical health and life expectancy disparities (Courtenay, 2011). Most recently, men in high positions in the media and corporate world, who thought they might be insulated from the changing rules, have been taken to task for exploiting their power relationships with women (Taub, 2017).

Changing norms in female self-expression and assertiveness have forced men to make an adjustment in their behaviors and expectations around control and power in their relationships. No longer is it acceptable to be abusive and controlling as a way to settle relational issues. Men require better interpersonal conflict skills. Unfortunately, many of the men with whom I have worked over the years have had difficulty shifting toward an egalitarian interpersonal dynamic with women.

Men's stress levels are further symptoms of change. With increased pressure and conflict at work and home, many men have sought refuge from the emotional intensity. Typical escape routes include overindulgence in food, alcohol, drugs, smoking, sex, and even work itself. Because traditional norms do not include men sharing their stress with others, men's psychological symptoms are often masked (Cochran & Rabinowitz, 2000). As long as it is "unmanly" to acknowledge anxiety and depression, these conditions eat away at men privately.

Today the rates of health-related medical conditions for men, especially cancers, cardiac problems, and diabetes, are higher in relation to rates for females (Gough & Robertson, 2017). Deaths as a result of violence, as well as traffic and industrial accidental deaths, occur among men at 3 to 4 times the rate they do among women (Centers for Disease Control and Prevention, 2015). Despite a higher reported prevalence of depression for women overall (Bromet et al., 2011; Kessler et al., 2003), the male suicide rate, especially in middle-aged White men, is 4 times that of women in the United States (Centers for Disease Control and Prevention, 2015; Phillips, Robin, Nugent, & Idler, 2010). Thus, it seems clear that men do experience depression, but many are not reporting it, nor are they seeking treatment, leading to a higher incidence of suicide than would be expected (Cochran & Rabinowitz, 2000; Phillips et al., 2010). Taking into account between-group variance and cross-national data, the average life expectancy for men globally is 5 to 7 years less than for women (Gough & Robertson, 2017).

Of course, many men were also at a disadvantage, even under the old rules. Men of color; gay, transgender, and bisexual men; disabled men; and men who don't fit into the straight White norms portrayed in the media have often been relegated to the shadows of society (Kimmel, 2017). These men have found prejudice and hate at the intersection of their masculine identities. The liberation movements that began in the 1960s and 1970s exposed some of the pent-up frustration of many groups of people, including women; people of color; and lesbian, gay, bisexual, transgender, and queer individuals. However, public policies and the structure and output of cultural institutions have been generally slow to transform and often still reflect societal conflict about maintaining the previous socioeconomic and social order.

## TURNING THE TIDE

Despite the difficulty of the transition, some men have taken advantage of changing gender expectations to expand their behavioral and emotional repertoires. They have been liberated from the forced roles of traditional masculinity and freed to pursue interests, careers, and relationships that might not fit that model. Their relationship patterns have shifted to include more egalitarian power and division of labor within the family. More fathers are nurturing, supportive, and positive with their children. There is hope in the breakdown of roles that men can live more productive, meaningful, and healthier lives.

By becoming more self-aware, men can make healthier choices about how they live. By questioning the traditional masculine norms, men have a chance to be better, well-rounded people. They can live more cooperatively and with greater concern for others. Being in control or in charge can be one of many ego states rather than the only one that feels comfortable. Competition to do one's best can be internally driven rather than compelled by a fear of inadequacy or a need to feel superior than another person. Ideally, by being more flexible and whole, men might become less aggressive and less needy for external acknowledgment.

Many men are still conflicted about how to handle the changing roles, the churning emotions, and the mixed messages that society gives about being a man. The message conveyed in the United States and other countries, reinforced by certain political groups, professional sports, and the advertising of male-oriented products, is that the "macho" version of manhood is still the best. The admiration of the "winners," who make large amounts of money, win at sports, or have flawless muscular bodies, is still ever present. Although most men never attain those ideals, many are tortured by the failure to live up to the standards they have internalized. Since childhood, many boys have been taught not to act like "sissies" by their peers on the playground. Although a good number of boys are supported emotionally at home, their entry into the public sphere is rife with competition and jockeying for who best lives up to the masculine ideal of toughness and dominance (Kilmartin & Smiler, 2015).

On an individual level, life is a rough journey regardless of one's cultural upbringing. There will be universal problems. Parents get divorced. Kids move away from friends. Friends betray each other. Parents and grandparents die or become incapacitated. Some young men will make mistakes and get in trouble with the law. Some will become addicted to alcohol or drugs. Adult men lose their jobs. Some men will search for love and never find it. Others will love, commit, and marry. Most men will experience leaving or being left by someone they love. Men will become fathers of kids who have special needs or difficult lives. Even those men who initially dodge some of life's dilemmas will be hit with them later in their lives. They will experience physical injury, suffer pain, and contract serious diseases. Eventually all of us will be left to ponder our own mortality and meaning in life. So even if we were perfectly capable of handling all of life's problems, we would still be impacted psychologically and emotionally by the challenges of the journey.

Under the best of circumstances, most of us would benefit from human support, understanding, and empathy as we make our way through life. Some are fortunate to have this kind of support in their families or communities, but many do not. Most men will tough it out and find a myriad of work-arounds when the unpredictable comes their way. Because asking for help, especially from a therapist or psychologist, is often perceived as shameful, most men never make it to a clinician's office, where potential supportive assistance is readily available. When they do, it is usually a last resort (Addis & Mahalik, 2003).

## SIGNIFICANCE AND SCOPE OF THIS BOOK

This book describes a personal approach to working therapeutically with men. It takes into account an individual's internal dynamics, the influences of culture, and the power of intimate therapeutic connections to deepen a man's experience of himself and his relationships. As you read, you will be able to witness how various men feel, think, and change as they move through the

Deepening individual and group psychotherapy process. My commentary and questions accompany the journey of each man and his interactions within the group setting. I provide the reader with my reactions, formulations, and reasons for interventions.

I have written the book to be relevant in terms of the literature in the field of individual and group psychotherapy with men, but more important I have chosen to give you a very personal look at this work. In the spirit of Irvin Yalom, psychiatrist and writer, I have shared with you interactive dialogues, as well as my private thoughts as I work with each man in both individual and group.

The book is organized to allow you to move from more general ideas and literature about men and therapy to the specifics of witnessing individual and group sessions. Part I includes background information on the Deepening Psychotherapy With Men model, as well as chapters on the principles of engaging men in individual therapy, the basics of group therapy as an approach, and what is unique and relevant about a men's therapy group. Part II highlights the individual therapy work and unique stories of the 10 men who will take part in the group therapy sessions described later. The chapters in Part II are written to give you both the background and a sense of how these men tell their stories, and how I as the therapist interact with and understand them. In each of these chapters, I emphasize the core issues each man is encountering, let you know why I believe the man would make a good group member, and ask you to reflect on the clinical issues raised in the sessions. In Part III, I lead you through a yearlong men's group that employs the principles of Deepening psychotherapy. These chapters, organized by the stage of the group, highlight dialog, developing relationships, and my perspective on the interventions and their impact. I also highlight practical tips for clinicians at the end of each of the group sessions. The final chapter answers questions about starting a men's group for your practice.

To protect confidentiality, all of the characteristics and names of the men depicted in the book have been significantly altered so that they are non-identifiable. The issues described are based on composites of individuals I have seen in my practice.

## MY JOURNEY: WHY THIS BOOK TAKES A PERSONAL APPROACH

For more than 35 years, I have acted as a guide to help men deepen their experience of themselves and one another. Far from being draining, it has been exciting, enlivening, and personally gratifying. I have learned much from those I have been privileged to join in their therapeutic journeys. I hope my experiences and scholarship can offer clinicians working with men a foundation for innovation in their approaches. If you are a practicing psychotherapist who is looking for new insights, or a graduate student trainee new to working with men, this book is for you.

I have written this book in a very personal way because it represents a significant aspect of my journey as a man and psychotherapist. I believe that men are hungry to tell their stories but often feel ashamed of the messiness they encounter as they take on real life. Instead of thinking that we must always have it "together," my assumption is that we all have to learn through our life experiences, including interactions with significant others, engaging in the world of school and work, and our attempts at finding meaning in the world. Often this means making mistakes, failing, and starting over. For me to encourage others to share their stories, I too must share mine. Although I may be a psychotherapist, I am also a fellow life traveler who has had to confront my own obstacles. Throughout the book, I reveal some of my own experiences as they are activated by the therapeutic work. It is my belief that exploring one's own depth is a prerequisite to facilitating this in others.

## THAWING MY OWN "ICE MAN" THROUGH THERAPY

Many of the men who come to see me seem encased in the restrictive cultural ice of what it means to be a man. I am no stranger to the metaphorical "Ice Man" (Rabinowitz, 2006). I know what it feels like to be barren and frozen in the realm of emotional expression. In my early life journey, I did catch glimpses of a possible "whole" self while high on drugs or in an alcohol-induced altered state of consciousness. I moved like a magnet toward emotionally intense women, hoping they would melt away my inner barrier to feeling. It was not until I gave in to the fact that I could not break free without help that I started to face my fear of what it meant to know my inner world.

My first therapy experience came in the fall after I graduated from college. I lacked direction. I felt trapped between depending on my well-meaning parents and my ex-girlfriend. I was afraid of being alone, yet I knew that none of these options felt right for me.

I committed to engaging in an in-depth self-analysis to learn how I had gotten to this stuck place. I was trapped by my demons of wanting others to accept and validate me, when I couldn't do this for myself. I had to undress my fears of being too vulnerable and dependent. My iced exterior needed some heat from a psychotherapist, who did not know me in any other way. I hated having to go through this process but knew that I could not go on living a frozen, hidden life. I dreamed of being successful, but there was no way I was going to be the alive, engaged, spontaneous person I wished I could be without this painful undressing.

It was very uncomfortable, mainly because of my own built-in prejudices about going to therapy. I told myself that it must mean there is something really wrong with me, and I didn't want to acknowledge I might be a defective human being. My first experience in treatment was with a female family systems therapist who was focused on my family dynamics. I initially resisted dismantling the narrative I had constructed about my mother and father as relatively flawless human beings, but eventually I opened my eyes to our family history and how I fit in the model. I realized that my high need for approval and achievement orientation was adaptive for me and our family narrative of success. The side effect of being this way was excessive worry, fear of failure, and not being comfortable in my own skin.

Something different happened when I encountered a male therapist who seemed to focus more on understanding me as a man. His approach took into account my male socialization and left me with less self-loathing and more appreciation for both the benefits and liabilities of my upbringing.

As a part of my journey toward becoming a therapist and better understanding myself, I sought out various types of therapy. I spent a couple of years recording all of my dreams for weekly Jungian analytic therapy. Unexpectedly, talking about the meaning of my dreams was more powerful than I could have ever imagined. I regularly found deep wisdom in my nightly adventures that often led to tears in my analyst's office as we reviewed their meaning. In Gestalt therapy, I learned to be very present with my emotions, acting them out with exaggerated movements and often voicing my contradictions by speaking to various aspects of myself. I found that I could give voices to my little boy, my judge, and my ideal self, as well as my fears about trusting my own hopes and desires. I spent time in bioenergetics therapy, learning to listen more to my body and how it manifested many of my psychological conflicts. I went to couples therapy to work on my failing marriage, only to learn that both of us had contributed to the destructive dynamic that doomed our long-term viability. And of course, I have been a part of many men's therapy experiences both as a participant and leader. Learning to trust other men with my inner thoughts and emotions was perhaps one of the most important lessons I have taken in. To feel supported and realize that I was not alone in my questioning of the values I was supposed to embrace as a man was liberating and made me even more committed to my work with men as a psychotherapist.

The ice has become less thick. I trust my inner compass more. I seek out personal growth experiences and know how to tolerate and embrace the discomfort that comes with outside feedback and new learning. Being able to be open, take risks, and be genuine in my interactions has turned out to be a lifetime journey, but I wouldn't want it any other way.

It is my hope that this book inspires you to do exciting clinical work with men but also to look inward and reflect on what you can learn as you follow the therapeutic journeys of those I describe in the book.

# I

# INDIVIDUAL AND GROUP PSYCHOTHERAPY WITH MEN

## INTRODUCTION: INDIVIDUAL AND GROUP PSYCHOTHERAPY WITH MEN

In order to best conceptualize how to work with men in Deepening psychotherapy, background information on the theory and practice is imperative. To that end, the first chapter in Part I highlights the Deepening psychotherapy with men model, highlighting the conflict zones that provide a structure for therapeutic intervention (Rabinowitz & Cochran, 2002). The model is based on an integration of the object relations and gender role strain paradigms, which also includes the intersectionality of nondominant culture influences. The conflict zones represent core issues that most men must face in their development and include ambivalence about relational dependence, confronting loss and grief, navigating dominant masculine self-structures, and a tendency to rely on doing over being when facing emotional conflict. The Deepening therapy model encourages the clinician to enter a man's depth portal by exploring emotional wounds that often have brought him to therapy.

The second chapter reviews ways that clinicians can enhance the chances of psychotherapy working with men. These include being aware of a man's stage of readiness and of ways to make the therapy experience more male-friendly and congruent with a man's socialization. By being sensitive to a man's ambivalence about seeking help based on his socialization, by mirroring his language and using relevant metaphors, and by using more self-disclosure, the therapy process with men is enhanced.

The third chapter reviews the basic principles of group psychotherapy, including the psychological benefits of group participation. By attending to how to create a safe environment, what effective group leaders do in practice, and the characteristics of the stages of group process, clinicians can identify the basic principles of a successful psychotherapy group.

In Chapter 4, the unique aspects of a men's psychotherapy group are described. These involve how to create trust among men who have been socialized to compete, what themes are likely to arise in discussion, characteristics of the group stages, and which interventions might best address the Deepening conflict zones that come up in the group setting.

# 1

# The Deepening Psychotherapy With Men Model

## *Identifying the Conflict Zones*

The Deepening approach to working with men was detailed in the book *Deepening Psychotherapy With Men* (Rabinowitz & Cochran, 2002) and was the result of extended observations of work with male clients, a thorough reading of the literature, and many long hours of discussion with my coauthor, Sam Cochran, about the psychodynamics of men, which had begun when we were in graduate school. We had initiated a men's group in 1981 at the University of Missouri, almost 10 years before Robert Bly (1990) wrote his popular mythopoetic look at masculinity, *Iron John*, and Sam Keen (1992) his seminal men's treatise, *Fire in the Belly: On Being a Man*. The combination of our graduate study in counseling psychology, our seeking a more thorough understanding of ourselves, and our desire to help struggling men propelled us to grapple with the seemingly difficult task of how to tap the male emotional depth we knew was there but was not often seen or valued. This first chapter provides a review of this paradigm.

Deepening therapy is characterized by the client and therapist jointly entering this wound portal to navigate the fears, defenses, and cultural gender role obstacles that have kept the inner emotional landscape from being owned and understood. The result of this exploration is a reconnection with a man's emotional world and an ensuing increase in self-expression and energy for life's activities (Rabinowitz & Cochran, 2002). Although there have not been clinical trials specific to the Deepening psychotherapy approach, many aspects of the described therapy process have been confirmed by clinicians who work with men. The relationship process variables have been recognized as the

http://dx.doi.org/10.1037/0000132-002
*Deepening Group Psychotherapy With Men: Stories and Insights for the Journey*,
by F. E. Rabinowitz

most significant aspect of psychotherapy outcome (Norcross & Lambert, 2011) and include approaching men with compassion, empathy, and positive regard, as well as entering each therapeutic relationship with nonjudgmental support to create a strong working alliance (Brooks, 2017).

The Deepening approach assumes that men have an emotional depth that can be uncovered, explored, and used to expand emotional and behavioral repertoires. The approach helps clinicians identify the conflict zones that their male clients must navigate in the journey toward greater psychological functioning. These zones, extracted from an integration of object relations and gender role strain theoretical perspectives, include ambivalence about relational dependence, the management of grief and loss, restrictive masculine self-structures, and the preference for "doing" over "being." Deepening psychotherapy itself involves identifying a man's depth portal, an opening into the deeper, emotional aspects of the self that is the result of the emotional wounding that has brought him to therapy (Rabinowitz & Cochran, 2002).

At its conceptual core, the Deepening approach to psychotherapy with men uses two major theoretical models to understand how men develop emotionally across the life span. The object relations perspective, a variant of the developmental psychodynamic approach, is based on observations of the early interaction of the child with parents and caretakers (Ainsworth, 1969). The gender role strain viewpoint identifies how the culture influences and reinforces the construction of roles that males are expected to enact. It takes into account dominant social norms as well as the intersection of nondominant cultural influences of the male experience. Although historically these two conceptualizations have been at odds with each other, their integration seems essential for understanding the inner emotional life of boys and men, and the manifestation of masculine identities within the wider culture (Rabinowitz & Cochran, 2002).

## AN OBJECT RELATIONS FORMULATION OF EARLY MALE DEVELOPMENT

Object relations theorists postulate that individual identity, that "sense of self" comprising a gendered component, develops from the complex interplay between the developing child and those other significant persons who make up the child's interpersonal milieu (Ainsworth, 1969). Early British object relations theorists focused on the developing child's attachment and separation from his primary caretakers (Bowlby, 1988). Winnicott (1988) suggested that "good enough" mothering through physical and emotional "holding" of the infant would provide optimal psychological development and integration. Bowlby (1988) and Mahler, Pine, and Bergman (1975) described the developmental tasks required of a child to move from dependence to independence, which included stages of oscillation between the two. The development of a gendered self occurred within the context of these close interpersonal relationships with first the mother and father and later with other important persons in the child's interpersonal milieu. These deeply personal, unique, and emotionally charged relationships provide the basis for the development of the boy's conception of what it means to be a boy and later inform his notions of what it means to be a man (Rabinowitz & Cochran, 2002). The mother, father, or primary caretaker who has developed his or her own idiosyncratic notions about the meaning of gender conveys expectations about a gendered self through interactions with the developing child.

Chodorow (1978) stated that gender is communicated interpersonally from the mother, when she is the primary caretaker:

> The different length and quality of the pre-oedipal period in boys and girls are rooted in women's mothering, specifically in the fact that a mother is of the same gender as her daughter and of a different gender from her son. This leads to her experiencing and treating them differently. (p. 98)

Chodorow argued that little boys experience a gender-specific "relational discontinuity" in their developmental progression from attachment through separation within the mother–child dyad. In contrast to little girls, who experience a connective sameness with the maternal figure that results in a joining of identity and relationship, little boys experience a sense of separateness as a part of their identity (Rabinowitz & Cochran, 2002).

Although Chodorow's (1978) analysis referred to the integration of cultural values, attachment, and gender identity in early life, Pollack (1995) postulated that perhaps little boys are pushed from connection to their mothers at an early age in conformity with our cultural values related to masculine independence. It is possible that little boys experience this push from the maternal orbit as a deep loss. Such an abrupt, often premature, separation experience is viewed as a

> traumatic abrogation of the early holding environment, an impingement in [a] boy's development—a normative life-cycle loss—that may, later in life, leave many adult men at risk for fears of intimate connection. This traumatic experience of abandonment occurs so early in the life course that the shameful memory of the loss is likely to be deeply repressed. (Pollack, 1995, p. 41)

Little boys' experience of the loss of maternal "holding" is thought to result in a self-protective, defensive firming of ego boundaries as well as internalized conflicts related to relationships and dependency (Rabinowitz & Cochran, 2002). The emotional aspect of this earliest inner experience of little boys' sense of self and other is "a normative male, gender-linked loss, a trauma of abandonment for boys which may show itself, later, as an adult through symptomatic behavior, characterological defense, and vulnerability to depression" (Pollack, 1998, p. 154).

This relatively common developmental trauma of separating prematurely from the maternal orbit will have a significant influence on the boy's evolving sense of self if it occurs early in his life. It is likely to result in a breakdown of empathic holding and a vulnerability to developing narcissistic-like compensating self-structures (Cochran & Rabinowitz, 1996; Pollack, 2005). To the extent that such developmental trauma is "normative" for boys, they are as a group more likely to have character structures distinguished by a firming of self-other boundaries, conflicts around dependency and relatedness, and an overvaluing of autonomy in service of preserving these structures (Rabinowitz & Cochran, 2002).

## THE GENDER ROLE STRAIN MODEL

The most researched analysis about gender role identity in boys and men comes from the study of the impact of cultural socialization. Gender roles are not biologically determined but rather are the enacted performances reinforced by society to maintain its social and economic order (Levant & Powell, 2017). The gender role strain paradigm suggests that the violation of gender role norms leads to social condemnation and negative psychological consequences for those who have internalized their value (Pleck, 1995). Men are thought to pay a steep emotional price for not following these norms, resulting in conformity, even when the roles are not healthy or adaptive (Pleck, 1981).

It has been suggested that the historical origins of masculine socialization are based on the training of boys and men to be hunters and warriors (Gilmore, 1991). David and Brannon (1976) coined the four preeminent values of Western culture's version of masculinity: "the big wheel," "the sturdy oak," "give 'em hell," and "no sissy stuff." The value of being a big wheel is embodied in being successful, important, and in charge. The significance of being a sturdy oak is portrayed in the masculine ideals of being tough, self-reliant, and confident. Give 'em hell means to be aggressive, competitive, and powerful both on the playing field and off. No sissy stuff requires restraining from showing affection, emotion, or any behavior that might be construed as feminine. Recent cross-cultural research studying the gender role socialization of Japanese men verifies adherence to the norms described by David and Brannon (Chan & Hayashi, 2010).

Underlying much of the male ideal has been an antifeminine stance. "You look like/you act like . . . a girl" is one of the shame-oriented put-downs that seems to have inhibited many boys from being more emotionally expressive. This has also translated into sanctioned homophobia that creates fear in men to touch or be verbally intimate with one another for fear of being identified as "gay." Even sensitive men are expected to publicly adhere to norms that reflect a male warrior culture that values power, control, aggression, and assertive heterosexual desire (Fenell, 2014; Kimmel, 2017).

In response to the civil rights, women's rights, and antiwar movements of the 1960s and 1970s, traditional rules and values of what was considered feminine and masculine came under attack. Our culture was changing, and men were challenged to respond to the contradictions of current and historical versions of masculinity. Although men were still being raised to be tough, strong, and powerful by our social institutions, they were also being asked to be more relational and sensitive by the women in their lives. Goldberg (1976),

Fasteau (1974), and Farrell (1975) were among the first writers to describe these binds and their confusing psychological consequences.

The study of men socialized with traditional masculine norms led to prolific research around the concept of gender role conflict. Gender role conflict is defined as "a psychological state in which socialized gender roles have negative consequences for the person or others. It occurs when rigid, sexist, or restrictive gender roles result in personal restriction, devaluation, or violation of others or oneself" (O'Neil, 2015, p. 42). O'Neil (2015) showed that gender role conflict was not a monolithic experience but rather occurred in the cognitive, emotional, behavioral, and unconscious domains in varying intrapersonal and interpersonal situations. His model has been the basis for numerous empirical studies that link a fear of femininity and the endorsement of traditional masculine ideology to restrictive emotionality; restrictive affectionate behavior between men; success, power, and competition issues; and conflicts between work and family (O'Neil, 2008). Continued research has shown that the endorsement of items that reflect a high degree of gender role conflict are correlated to higher levels of psychological distress, including depression (i.e., Shepard, 2002), alcohol and substance abuse (i.e., Monk & Ricciardelli, 2003), aggression (i.e., Cohn & Zeichner, 2006), low self-esteem (i.e., Mahalik, Locke, Theodore, Cournoyer, & Lloyd, 2001), and avoidance of mental and physical health-care venues (i.e., Good, Dell, & Mintz, 1989).

Although today there appears to be some tolerance for variations in the masculine ideal in many subgroups of Western culture, many boys still grow up believing that they must follow what Pollack (1999) called the "boy code." They must be tough on the playground, keep their vulnerable emotions in check, restrict impulses toward expressing affection, and laugh or keep quiet when another boy is being victimized. This early restriction on emotion and self-expression leaves many men in adulthood with problematic communication skills and normative alexithymia. *Alexithymia* is defined as an inability to put words on emotions (Levant, 1998).

## ETHNICITY, CULTURE, AND GENDER IDENTITY INTERSECTIONS

Ethnic and cultural identity intersect powerfully with gender role influences to shape masculine expectations about how to act and conceive of oneself. For many men of color who grow up outside mainstream European American, heterosexual, middle-class culture, they are reminded by their experiences of prejudice and oppression on a personal and institutional level that although they are men, they are less privileged and more vulnerable to forces outside of their control (Caldwell & White, 2005).

Although many men try to maintain a color-blind perspective, America is still racially divided. Even with the recent incidents of shootings of Black men and the protests generated by Black Lives Matter, it is still difficult for White men to comprehend the subtle harassment that men of color experience on a daily basis. Questionable stares, increased scrutiny, and automatic suspicion by peers, strangers, and police are regular occurrences for these men who work and live in the mainstream culture (Barry, Kovaleski, Robertson, & Alvarez, 2012; Majors & Gordon, 1994; Winter & Vallano, 2016). Not only are they subject to the stresses of traditional masculinity, they must also cope with the overlay of subtle and not-so-subtle racism. A layer of frustration that can manifest as anger or depression related to this cultural predicament is common in many men of color, even those who are trying to live by the rules of mainstream society (Franklin, 1998).

Although not as obvious as skin color, there are varieties of "White" identity as well that leave men vulnerable to feelings of alienation. Men who are unemployed or who work in the blue-collar work sector may feel alienated from those in white-collar jobs. In many places in America, gay men are fearful of expressing aspects of their sexual orientation in the presence of their straight counterparts. Transgender men are especially vulnerable to prejudice and misunderstanding but also susceptible to mental health distress that few clinicians are trained to address (American Psychological Association, 2015). Jews, Muslims, Christians, and men from other religious backgrounds also feel ambivalence about how public they should be in acknowledging their religious identities. Men with physical and psychological disabilities can be subject to unwanted scrutiny and judgment from other men. Men struggling with issues of underemployment or unemployment may present with defensiveness that belies underlying fears of being judged for not living up to perceived masculine ideals. For most men, not only is there strain from trying to adhere to traditional gender role norms but also the added stress of being true to one's unique version of masculine identity.

## INTEGRATING OBJECT RELATIONS AND GENDER ROLE STRAIN: THE DEEPENING CONFLICT ZONES

The integration of the object relations and gender role strain models conveys the unfolding of an individually constituted, interpersonally related masculinity with the influences of cultural norms. This integration offers both insight into and empathy for men's psychological development. It brings in the power of the cultural milieu into the developmental process. Therapists, working with both of these perspectives to guide them, can increase their empathy for men's difficulties, have greater clinical resonance with men's struggles, and will thereby have greater conceptual clarity to inform their therapeutic practices with men (Rabinowitz & Cochran, 2002).

Highlights from these models can be organized into conflict zones that the Deepening therapist can use to understand how a man has been impacted and how to guide the therapy process. These conflict zones include ambivalence about relational dependence; prohibition against sadness, grief, and mourning; problematic masculine-specific self-structures; preferences for doing instead of being; and the emotional wounding that has brought a man to therapy (Rabinowitz & Cochran, 2002).

### Ambivalence About Relational Dependence

Masculinity in contemporary American culture emphasizes independence, the capacity to "stand on your own two feet," and all that is associated with this particular psychological value. How does the developing little boy, who is initially unaware of the way his culture devalues his dependence, negotiate this experience? How does our culture's ambivalence about, and disavowal of, dependency in males become integrated into boys' and men's psychological lives? The little boy is dependent on his early caretakers for feeding, holding, and shelter, as well as love and support. This is a universal human developmental experience, yet in the messages that dominate our American culture, dependence and its psychological meaning are often seen as contraindicated with masculinity. This early relationship with a caretaker, characterized by dependence, longing, and (it is hoped) gratification, forms the basis for expectations in boys' and men's relationships with their own mothers, and later with both men and women in their lives (Rabinowitz & Cochran, 2002).

Often, the longing and gratification that the little boy experiences are culturally devalued as he grows into manhood. Males are confronted by cultural messages that they are unmanly and abnormal if they experience gratification from their dependency needs. Boys are prone to internalize contradictory, mixed interpretations of their experience because of their underlying ambivalence about dependency. On one hand, they experience affirmation and gratification of dependency in their early relations with mother and other important adults. On the other hand, they learn that such an experience is to be disavowed if they are to be accepted as a male. Other powerful forces in the social landscape that may also reinforce this learning include parents, teachers, coaches, and especially same-sex peers.

Disapproval and shame become associated with the presence and enactment of dependency needs. To disavow the most basic of psychological needs—the need to depend on another person for love, support, and nurturance—results in a boy or man who must "stand on his own two feet" and not ask for help or support, even under the most disturbing circumstances. It also may result in a distancing in interpersonal relationships so as not to appear needy or dependent. Pollack (1998) called this *defensive autonomy*. In intimate relationships, it might manifest as an avoidance of emotional intensity or an unwillingness to commit out of fear of being engulfed.

In the therapeutic relationship, the conflict about dependence manifests itself in several ways. The fact that few men even make it to a therapist reflects the avoidance of men in our culture of involving themselves in a potentially dependent relationship, even if it is for their own good. Another demonstration of this conflict results in the devaluing of the therapeutic relationship, particularly early in the process. Men in the initial stages of therapy often perceive it more as an impersonal psychological "tune-up" rather than an intimate relational process. The dependence conflict may also be manifest as a perceived lack of commitment by the male client to the therapeutic endeavor (Rabinowitz & Cochran, 2002).

Sometimes therapists misinterpret a man's closed posture, simple and gruff language, hesitancy to share, and lack of emotional expression as resistance that needs to be overcome rather than an expression of the conflicting nature of dependent urges toward the therapist and therapy. The roots of this dilemma lie deep for many men. Basic ambivalence around dependence and intimacy played out in a relational context recapitulates the earliest experiences of dependency and relational "holding" with the mother and father. Adult intimacy is often associated with vulnerability and, ultimately, with disconnection; the man unconsciously remembers his connection—then disconnection—with his earliest love object. The "blank" that many men draw when asked for deeper commitment may be the present-day enactment of this early relational conundrum (Rabinowitz & Cochran, 2002).

### Prohibitions Against Sadness, Grief, and Mourning

From an early age, little boys are presented with both overt and covert messages suggesting that they suppress their emotional experience and their expression of feelings. "Crybaby," "keep a stiff upper lip," "man up," and "gut it out" are but a few of the admonitions given to little boys to deny, disavow, and suppress outward expression of their sad or vulnerable emotions. Such values expressed by parents and other caretakers profoundly shape the growing boy's interpretation of his experience of loss and grief and have a long-lasting impact on the manner by which he eventually learns to mourn his losses. This is particularly problematic in light of the fact that both boys and girls experience disappointments, betrayals, and losses from birth onward. Just as girls and women are often perceived to be more comfortable with these emotions, boys and men seem alarmed by them. As a result, boys and men frequently dissociate themselves from these feelings and repress them deep into the hidden realms of their inner lives.

Dissociation, as a defensive psychological process, can compromise the natural mourning that occurs as a result of the making and breaking of intimate emotional attachments to others throughout the life span. When this normal process of grieving is truncated and thrown off course, anger, shame, and control-oriented defenses often arise as a means of self-protection. This also creates conditions that invite self-medication and acting out to relieve the discomfort caused when these emotions threaten to break through into consciousness. Perhaps it is through this dynamic that we can understand why so many men suffer from alcohol and substance abuse problems and tend to "distract" or act out many of their emotions in both benign and destructive ways (Cochran & Rabinowitz, 2000; Rabinowitz & Cochran, 2008).

In the therapeutic relationship, issues of grief and loss and the accompanying emotional experience of sadness may be elusive or difficult to acknowledge.

A male client may describe a loss experience and take a "what can I do about it now?" attitude instead of moving toward the emotional level of experiencing the loss. Similarly, a male client may minimize the impact of a loss experience, saying, "It's no big deal, I can handle this." Often when a therapist openly addresses loss and grief issues, many men find a new and rich level of emotional experience (Cochran, 2005; Cochran & Rabinowitz, 1996). Therapy that encourages male clients to talk about loss experiences can facilitate the unclogging of the emotional ice jam that has been maintained by shame and the fear of losing control.

## Problematic Masculine-Specific Self Structures

As a result of contemporary child-rearing practices and the influence of relationships with siblings, peers, teachers, and the popular media, a boy's psychological development is intimately intertwined with conscious and unconscious transmissions of cultural values around masculinity and femininity. Little boys are given mixed and incongruous messages about how important others view their masculinity. Such messages often conflict with their inner experiences of emotional need and desire. The development of a coherent sense of self with a positively valued facet of masculinity is therefore a significant challenge for many boys. As many boys venture into puberty, problematic aspects of their masculinity have been well learned and suppressed, resulting in a flattening of the emotional expression of sadness, anguish, fear, and tenderness. At the same time, many male adolescents tend toward acting out emotional conflict through risk taking and aggressiveness (Cochran & Rabinowitz, 2000).

As boys begin to construct masculine-specific self-structures, they must balance how peers, family, and the cultural influences of school and the media view certain aspects of masculinity with their own acquisition of masculine traits. Often, these outer definitions of masculinity conflict with inner needs, wishes, and values. The boy, who is hurt and needs emotional support, or even a hug, is sometimes admonished to "stop crying" and "take it like a man." Over time, such contradictory and mixed admonitions result in the creation of a facade of problematic masculine-specific self-structures designed to hide vulnerability and apparent weakness. Such self-structures include a tendency to restrict emotional awareness and expression, a propensity to distance or withdraw from interpersonal connection, a discomfort with depressive feelings and the corresponding expression through tears, and a penchant to show force or action when encountering a personal problem (Rabinowitz & Cochran, 2002).

Conflicting masculine self-structures are often one of the reasons a man may come to therapy. The denial of sadness and loss, the retreat from intimacy in relationships, compulsive competitiveness, the neglect of physical and emotional health, and other "traditional" masculine ways of being often have detrimental consequences to the man as well as his relationships with those he loves. Understanding the conditions under which these self-structures have been created and working on dismantling the dysfunctional elements is an important therapeutic focus of gender-sensitive psychotherapy for men.

### Preferences for "Doing" Versus "Being"

In observing a typical school playground, one might notice that boys are often involved in competitive, active play within larger groups. Girls are frequently involved in smaller groups of more relational, cooperative play. These sex differences appear to persist into adulthood and are thought to reflect externalizing defense styles (Gjerde, Block, & Block, 1988), distracting response styles (Nolen-Hoeksema, 1990), or externalizing ego defenses (Levit, 1991).

Winnicott (1988) believed that *being* was a universal developmental milestone accomplished by the union of a "good enough" environmental (maternal/paternal) adaptation with the infant's physical and emotional needs. It is out of this elementary experience of being held and nurtured that the capacity for true *doing* arises. *Doing* corresponds to the spontaneous, joyful emergence of the "real self" and the actions taken to activate and outwardly express this self. Such behavior is based on—or evolves out of—the basic capacity for simply *being* that is characterized by an absence of restlessness and contentment with one's emotional self. Despite believing that both men and women can experience both states, Winnicott noted that girls and women seemed to be more comfortable with being and boys and men more at home with doing.

Boys' preference for doing over being can be observed in a number of ways. As noted, the little boy may prefer active, physical play on the playground with his friends at an early age. In addition, boys and men appear to prefer more action-oriented means of problem solving that may have adaptive as well as maladaptive consequences. Adaptive doing is seen in active problem solving, a willingness to take risks to protect others, and a capacity for hard work that characterize many men. Maladaptive doing is observed in unseemly risk taking, difficulty relaxing, and/or overt and destructive acting-out behaviors that often serve as distractions from unpleasant emotional states. Aggression and problems with various kinds of addictions from substance abuse to compulsive gambling to sexual promiscuity to workaholism are also forms of maladaptive doing (Rabinowitz & Cochran, 2002).

Men's tendency for doing, and a discomfort for being, can be seen as a relevant component of many men's emotional and relational difficulties. As the unpleasant and destructive consequences of a life that is based on an over-reliance on doing accrue, therapists can help men recognize the value in cultivating their capacity for being and strive to strike a balance between doing and being. Relational bonds that have occurred through productive doing can be strengthened by a therapeutic approach that intertwines activity in the therapy relationship along with a focus on being with the feelings that emerge. The familiar doing approach can often act as an entryway to the being world. With an appreciation of the meaning of both of these elements for men, a sensitive psychotherapist may be better able to facilitate the attainment of this balance.

## THE WOUND AS A PORTAL TO UNDERSTANDING A MAN'S DEPTH

Most, if not all, problems that men present to a psychotherapist have an element of wounding. *Wounding* refers here to the nature of the experience that has precipitated a visit to the therapist. Interpersonal conflict and rejection, failure experiences, and frustrations with not meeting expectations of life all can be construed as wounding experiences for many men. Deaths of family and friends, the inevitable confrontation with aging and physical decline, or the reconciliation of one's life dreams with reality's limitations are often felt as wounds to men (Rabinowitz & Cochran, 2002).

Wounds challenge a man's basic sense of self. They bring to awareness a man's shortcomings, or his perceived failure to live up to his culture's masculine ideals. Such perceptions are felt as failure and are, as such, experienced as a "narcissistic wound" to the ego (Kohut, 1977). A rejection in an intimate relationship has an obvious element of wounding. The man who is rejected often enters therapy feeling confused, hurt, angry, and unable to understand completely what may have "gone wrong." The man's sense of adequacy as a partner, both sexual and social, has been challenged. His view of himself must be reconciled with his partner's view of himself. The realignment of self-perception and another's perception is frequently a painful one for many men.

Failure at work is a similar wounding. A man who is fired or laid off from his job experiences a sense of failure and inadequacy. A process of realignment, similar to that which occurs with rejection in an intimate relationship, takes place wherein the man must reconcile his own perceptions with others' perceptions. In addition, his identity as a provider is challenged. Deepening therapy is characterized by the client and therapist jointly entering this wound portal to navigate the fears, defenses, and cultural gender role obstacles that have kept the inner emotional landscape from being owned and understood. The result of this exploration is a reconnection with a man's emotional world and an ensuing increase in self-expression and energy for life's activities (Rabinowitz & Cochran, 2002).

# 2

# Making Psychotherapy Work for Men

It is not often that men seek a counselor or therapist willingly. The stigma associated with seeking help acts as a barrier for men (Vogel, Heimerdinger-Edwards, Hammer, & Hubbard, 2011). More likely, men look for help as a result of an ultimatum by a partner or family member or a mandate from legal authorities. Often the breakthrough behavior that triggers encouragement to seek help comes as a result of not knowing how to cope effectively with trauma, loss, addiction, depression, or illness (Rabinowitz, 2014a). Men who feel coerced into therapy often arrive uncomfortable and defensive upon entry (Brooks, 2017). A smaller percentage of men choose the psychotherapeutic path willingly as a result of a previous therapy or support group experience or as an educational venture to extend self-learning that had previously been awakened (Rabinowitz & Cochran, 2002).

Epidemiological surveys suggest that the most widely reported mental health problems for men involve alcohol and drug use/dependency (Kessler et al., 2003). Less prevalent but significant are depression, social phobia, and antisocial personality disorder. Cochran and Rabinowitz (2000) speculated that for many men, the shame of portraying oneself as weak, sad, or confused leads to a masking of their inner turmoil. By adhering to the traditional masculine self-structures, like restricting overt emotionality, acting powerful and strong, and being self-reliant, men leave themselves few outlets for dealing with dysphoric emotional states. The result might be silent withdrawal from close relationships, irritability or grumpiness, angry outbursts, or the intake of

http://dx.doi.org/10.1037/0000132-003
*Deepening Group Psychotherapy With Men: Stories and Insights for the Journey*,
by F. E. Rabinowitz

mood-altering substances (Cochran & Rabinowitz, 2000). Addis and Hoffman (2017) suggested that the norms of emotional control and self-reliance make it difficult for men to not only acknowledge their own emotional suffering but communicate it to others. Our culture has come to expect men to be inexpressive, further allowing them to hide behind their societal masks without question (Addis, 2011). A more sensitive diagnostic lens could potentially detect that not all is "all right" with men who are inexpressive or who enact the strong, self-reliant front, but usually they get a pass because they are not acting outside of normative behavioral parameters for males in society.

The men who are identified as needing some psychological help often have a "leaky" coping mechanism that is not working to contain inner turmoil. For instance, men who cannot contain their feelings of hopelessness get aggressive in their interactions with others, become belligerent when drinking alcohol, engage in high-risk activities such as driving too fast, participate in gambling that leads to money problems, or engage in compulsive sex may find that their lives are spinning out of control. A run-in with the law, broken interpersonal relationships, or financial difficulties may leave them exposed and potentially open to psychological intervention. In addition, men who have experienced loss or trauma may feel overwhelmed, with their normal coping mechanisms not up to the task of containing emotional distress. This suffering might include a significant relationship loss, a change in work identity, or a health crisis that makes it difficult to employ one's usual distracting tactics that minimize awareness and acknowledgment of agitated internal emotional states.

## READINESS FOR PSYCHOTHERAPY

Brooks (2010) has a matrix for male clients who come to therapy based on their readiness to engage in treatment. By using the precontemplation and action stages of change model (Prochaska & Norcross, 2003), as well as the coercive pressure being applied by outside forces, Brooks differentiated the goals of therapy, the tasks to be accomplished, and the nature of the therapeutic relationship.

The male client most resistant to change is the individual who has not questioned his own behavior and has little outside pressure to do so. Only occasionally do these men come to therapy. It has been my experience that a respected close friend, partner, or family member has made the suggestion that he attend, but the individual is really in a precontemplative stage, in which he doesn't quite know what to work on or why he really needs to be there. A therapist engaging this type of man needs to be more of an educator about how male gender role pressures may keep him from doing everything he might. Ideally, a therapist might hook a male client by talking about masculinity and its potential impact on one's life. It is not expected that the client will stay in treatment very long from this position, but by having an experience of therapy as a nonthreatening situation, this man might return in the future.

A rare but significant male client is the one who is ready to change but has very little environmental support for doing so (Brooks, 2010). In this case, the individual is feeling internal pressure to make a change but fears that in doing so he will upset the equilibrium of his support system. Joe, a police officer for the past 10 years, came to therapy because of his extreme sensitivity to the emotions of those in his environment. Joe grew up in a low socioeconomic neighborhood, excelled at school, and became a policeman when it was suggested by a respected teacher. Joe enjoyed the interpersonal aspects of the job but had grown increasingly troubled by the pain he could read on those with whom he had to interact, especially troubled teenagers. He was bothered by the cavalier and prejudicial attitudes of his colleagues. At home, Joe was also troubled by his wife's drinking and the disturbing interactions he had with his divorced parents. He felt that he had to be "the rock" for everyone, and it was getting to him. In this situation, the therapist validated Joe's concerns and emotional reactions. Joe appreciated having a place to talk about feeling overwhelmed, because his outside life left him few opportunities to be authentic. Joe was eventually referred to a men's therapy group, where his feelings could be expressed and understood without his having to worry about jeopardizing his job. Therapy also gave him a chance to work on changing the dynamics of his family relationships.

The most common male client is the one who is in the precontemplative stage of change but is being highly pressured to come to therapy by the environment (Brooks, 2010). Brooks (1998b) suggested a "soft-sell" approach to engagement in which the therapist acknowledges the resistance a man might have to being in treatment while building a strong therapeutic alliance. Brooks (2010) wrote,

> In the common situation in which a male client has been more or less coerced into therapy, a therapist is prudent to maximize the strategic benefits of the triangulated position. . . . For example, useful questions might be as follows: "What is it that your wife (boss, doctor, judge) is so worked up about?" "What do we need to do to get them off of your back?" From this position, the therapist can mediate the benevolently between the troubled factions without losing credibility with either. (p. 78)

In many ways, the therapist can thus ally himself or herself with the precontemplative male client and get him to begin to take ownership for the problems that others are noting without triggering resistance.

The male client who is ready to make changes and has the environmental support to do so is likely to require the least amount of direction from the therapist. Brooks (2010) suggested that the therapist act as an empathic, collaborative facilitator who encourages the male client to pursue his goals. The therapist in this scenario is more likely to be able to confront a male client when he is falling back into old patterns or is internally fearful of how change will affect his life.

## CREATING A MALE-FRIENDLY THERAPY ENVIRONMENT

Men in psychological pain who have been socialized to not ask for help are a challenge for the psychotherapist (Englar-Carlson & Stevens, 2006). Traditional talk psychotherapy, which relies on the individual experiencing distress to share his inner feelings with a caring clinician, is often not the model most men would endorse. Brooks (2017) argued that conventional psychotherapy that does not recognize gender socialization might be harming men by turning them off from seeing counseling as a viable option. The dilemma for therapists who want to be successful in helping many male clients, who may not be comfortable with the therapy situation, is how to shift their approach to be more male friendly.

### Empathy for Male Socialization

In response to the reluctance of men to make use of therapy, several authors have reconceptualized and adapted therapeutic methods to take into consideration the way men have been raised and interact in their everyday lives. At the core of most of these approaches is a requirement that clinicians do their best to educate themselves about how men construct their masculinity identity, individually and collectively (Englar-Carlson, Evans, & Duffey, 2014). By understanding cultural norms for men, a therapist can come into the encounter with a male client with compassion and empathy rather than judgment (Rabinowitz, 2006). From the decorum and reading material in the waiting area to the language a therapist uses, it is possible to make a statement that this therapeutic environment will be friendly, not foreign (Rabinowitz & Cochran, 2002). It goes a long way toward reducing initial anxiety and shame to acknowledge a man's ambivalence and courage when he first comes into the consulting room. An approach that focuses on male strengths (in contrast to flaws and weakness) has been shown to have a powerful effect on men's willingness to embrace the therapy experience (Englar-Carlson & Kiselica, 2013).

### Interest in a Man's Unique Identity

Because identity is not monolithic, it is important for clinicians to understand the intersection of variables that might have shaped a man's masculine self (Englar-Carlson et al., 2014). Race, ethnicity, age, sexual orientation, gender identity, cultural upbringing, education, socioeconomic standing, religious/spiritual affiliation, migration status, and ability status will impact how a man experiences his masculine identity (Wong, Liu, & Klann, 2017). Although a clinician might not know everything about each of these influential variations, being open, interested, and inquisitive to the uniqueness of the individual will encourage a man share more of himself (Nadal & Rivera, 2014).

The following exchange is a dialogue with Enrique, a Mexican American man in his early 30s who has come to therapy to work on feelings of low self-worth and depression. The therapist is probing to understand how the client sees himself as a man.

**THERAPIST:** So both of your parents worked long hours when you were young. How did that impact you?

**ENRIQUE:** I spent a lot of time watching my younger siblings. I rarely did any extracurricular activities since I had family responsibilities.

**THERAPIST:** So you had to be like a parent to your brother and sister?

**ENRIQUE:** Yes. It was expected. I felt like we had to keep a low profile, since my parents were migrant workers. I remember my mom telling me we shouldn't even play outside and draw attention to ourselves.

**THERAPIST:** Seems like you were forced to keep things low key and secret.

**ENRIQUE:** Looking back, it felt pretty restrictive. I never questioned it. I didn't want to cause my parents any more stress, since they seemed like they had all they could handle.

**THERAPIST:** So you tried your best to be good and responsible.

**ENRIQUE:** Yes. That sums me up except that inside I didn't feel good about myself. I had few friends at school and none that I ever could invite to my house. I didn't develop very good social skills. I was shy and awkward in public. Even when my father, who was a very proud man, would praise me, I felt like a fraud. I felt like I was playing a part to make him and my mom not feel guilty for working all the time. I never felt like I could tell them how I really felt.

**THERAPIST:** While you outwardly were very responsible, I sense that you carried around shame about who you were.

**ENRIQUE:** Yes. I think that may be some of the source of the feelings I carry with me now as an adult. I feel like I don't belong a lot of the time. It silences me. Who would want to hang out with me?

**THERAPIST:** I can sense that it is painful for you.

### Mirroring Language and Metaphor

By listening to the language, inflection, and vocabulary a man speaks, a clinician can adapt his or her interaction patterns to that particular client (Rabinowitz & Cochran, 2002). A strong part of the therapeutic alliance comes from the quality of the interpersonal communication. To believe that you "get him," a male client often needs to feel as if you are speaking a similar language. By noting the words he uses and using them in the conversation, a therapist can create an easier bond with a male client. The clinician's use of relevant metaphors that are based on the client's real-life experiences is another powerful tool that involves mirroring language and perspective (Rabinowitz & Cochran, 2002). Although some traditional therapists believe that metaphors are a way to intellectually distance from material, many men seem to resonate with metaphors as a way to express how they actually frame their felt experience (McKelley, 2014). Words that describe scenes or imagery seem to be readily applied to a man's emotional life. It is the language that has often seemed missing from the male vocabulary. It is a language of the outdoors and of objects. It fits with the more external, experiential orientation that many men have (Rabinowitz & Cochran, 2002). Because traditional male socialization minimizes a focus on feelings, pinpointing specific emotional states is often more difficult than finding equivalent action-oriented metaphors that convey a holistic sense of what is being experienced.

Lars, 20, came to therapy after he had been suspended from his university for being involved in a vandalism incident. Lars was severely intoxicated when he and a friend broke a window in a dorm room and were accused of stealing computer equipment. The following exchange is a therapeutic dialogue early in treatment that incorporates metaphor.

**THERAPIST:** What does it mean for you to be here right now?

**LARS:** I don't know. I still can't believe I did something so stupid. That's not who I am.

**THERAPIST:** Who are you?

**LARS:** You know, I am someone who was raised with good values. It's like I temporarily lost my compass.

**THERAPIST:** Lost your compass?

**LARS:** Yeah. I guess when I was drinking, it was like I was driving without GPS. I realize now that I have a definite problem with alcohol. I am sorry for what I did.

**THERAPIST:** You regret your actions because you really drove off the road this time.

**LARS:** Yes. There are some real consequences. Right now, I'm not sure if I can face anyone, my friends and especially my family. I have really let them down.

## Therapist Self-Disclosure

Another way that clinicians can increase the receptivity of male clients is through relevant and appropriate therapist self-disclosure (Wexler, 2014). Shame about asking for help and discomfort at being in an interpersonally demanding situation can be mitigated by a clinician sharing some of his or her humanness (Henretty & Levitt, 2010). Therapist small talk sharing about a local sports team at the beginning of a session to a relevant personal story in the context of a dilemma in the midst of a session can take away some of the perceived judgment a client may be feeling. Well-timed and relevant self-disclosure may act as a point of connection for a male client to feel as if he can let down some of his defenses.

Horace, 33, came to therapy to deal with relationship issues. His long-term girlfriend had recently left him. Much of his validation had come from her, and now he was beginning to realize that he would have to give this to himself. The following exchange is a therapeutic dialogue that reflects the use of self-disclosure.

**HORACE:** I wish I had seen this coming. Until she left, I did not realize how much I relied on her to define who I am.

**THERAPIST:** It seems like you are now left with just you to be with yourself.

**HORACE:** I know. I'm not that confident I have the tool set for this.

**THERAPIST:** When I was a younger man, I had a similar kind of breakup. It was really hard, but I learned a lot about myself.

**HORACE:** What did you learn? I could use some guidance.

**THERAPIST:** While my situation is not the same, I was forced to learn how to be my own friend.

**HORACE:** You mean give yourself your own feedback and trust it?

**THERAPIST:** Exactly.

**HORACE:** That is what I want to work on while I am here.

Regardless of the therapy approach, the working alliance is strengthened by sensitivity to the factors that predispose a man to be more comfortable in this intense interpersonal situation. By seeing the world through their client's eyes, clinicians can more easily make adjustments in language, reduce judgmental comments, and disclose relevant information that humanizes the encounter. The result is an increase in the willingness of a male client to share and be open to the give-and-take inherent in the therapy experience (Brooks, 2017).

# 3

# Group Therapy

## *The Why and How*

Almost all humans are raised in a variety of group environments, including family groups, friend groups, school classrooms, and work groups. In common public settings such as playgrounds, restaurants, and shopping malls, individuals from various backgrounds gather, mostly unaware of the social psychological dynamics that govern their interactions. The group is a familiar setting for human behavior but also one wrought with potential problems. Each group has its own social norms, cultural rules, and expectations of behavior. For some, this makes the group a place of safety, predictability, and structure, but for many it also brings potential shame, restriction on behavior, and imbalance, depending on the nature of its rules, hierarchies, and enforcement.

### WHY GROUP THERAPY?

As a therapeutic modality, group therapy will often recapitulate some of the group environments that many of us have encountered in our lives (Yalom & Leszcz, 2005). For those who have previously found solace in talking to others about our struggles, the group offers a receptive cadre of fellow life travelers. For those whose past group experiences were more painful, shaming, or restrictive, the group can represent a threatening environment of judgment and potential retraumatization. This may be especially true of individuals

http://dx.doi.org/10.1037/0000132-004
*Deepening Group Psychotherapy With Men: Stories and Insights for the Journey*,
by F. E. Rabinowitz

who do not share the physical, racial, sexual, or cultural norms of the majority culture (Kottler & Englar-Carlson, 2014). As a therapy process, group has been shown to provide effective support for individuals who struggle with similar concerns while acknowledging and addressing the fear and hesitation that has come as a result of negative life experiences (Burlingame, MacKenzie, & Straus, 2004).

The challenge for a group therapist is to create a space that is safe but capable of handling the potential anxiety, anger, and shame that many group members will feel when placed in this vulnerable setting. Some would argue that individual therapy removes these obstacles by having a one-to-one relationship with a trained psychotherapist who can empathize and assist without the triggers of other people present. A client might talk about painful episodes in a trusting space but not have to directly encounter the immediacy of perceived judgment or scrutiny by peers. The individual therapy experience provides some psychological distance to look at the issues and not be overwhelmed with emotion.

Except through transference or direct action by the therapist, individual therapy does not provide the present interpersonal stimuli that might lead to a here-and-now reexperiencing some of the individual's core concerns. Individual therapy also does not offer the multiple perspectives, feedback, and support of a number of interested observers. For instance, an individual listening to another member of the group talk about his father might think about his own relationship with his father, experience an emotional reaction to this memory, and then be directed by the therapist to share this with the other members. This disclosure might not only lead to a deeper exploration of this relationship but encourage others to talk more extensively about their fathers and provide supportive validation to the individual who initiated the discussion.

Potential clients need to be informed of what the group experience will be like so that they can make a thoughtful decision about whether it is right for them. Having previous individual counseling or therapy is often a useful precursor to understanding the language and intimacy required for sharing oneself in a group (Rabinowitz, 2014b). Individuals without therapy experience often need time to take in the rules of engagement in this environment. It can be helpful for the group leader to put together a booklet or handout about how to get the most from the group experience, how the interpersonal aspects of group might function, and explicit rules about confidentiality. Often a clinician who has worked one-on-one with a client will recommend that the client participate in a group to improve communication skills or to get additional support and feedback for a particular concern such as depression, divorce, or loss. It is not uncommon for this client to still check in regularly with the individual therapist, especially when psychological material from the group interactions touches long-standing core concerns in the individual.

## BENEFITS OF GROUP

For those ready for the experience, group therapy is a powerful approach that encourages learning from others in a psychologically focused and interpersonally monitored environment. Group provides a way for isolated participants to purposefully interact with one another to become more aware of their own behavior, to practice more effective relating, and to gain a wider and more universal perspective on their lives (Yalom & Leszcz, 2005). By encouraging feedback from members, individuals can gain new insights into their behavior and blind spots that may be sabotaging relationships in their lives. Group allows members to practice interpersonal relating and provides opportunities for vicarious learning through observing others in the group work on their issues. These lessons can then be applied outside the group setting when the individual is ready. Group therapy allows those being helped to also be helpers. The suggestions, feedback, and personal reactions to another member's concerns often lead to feelings of competence and helpfulness in those individuals. Effective interpersonally oriented groups often help members understand how their family of origin has impacted their current relationships. A long-term group that has fostered trust and intimacy can serve as a surrogate family, providing some of the qualities of a high-functioning family or community (Yalom & Leszcz, 2005).

Often, individuals in groups find that their thoughts, feelings, and perspectives are more universal than they had previously believed, providing a sense of comfort and support rather than the isolation many people feel in their everyday lives. In addition, group therapy encourages individuals to try to more deeply understand repeating patterns of behavior or difficult emotions in a supportive environment. An insight or decision to change a life pattern can often be more easily recalled and applied in the presence of witnesses. Perhaps most important, group therapy can instill hope in individuals that change and life improvement are possible (Yalom & Leszcz, 2005).

## MAKING GROUPS SAFE

Much of the effectiveness of group therapy depends on how the focus and structure of the group matches up with the issues and characteristics of the participants. Group therapists must have knowledge of how to create a trusting environment and how to handle the difficult situations that can arise that might cause harm to individuals in the group setting. Kottler and Englar-Carlson (2014) recommended that group therapists put into place protections against potential negative outcomes. Such protections include the following:

- Prepare all group participants before the first session for what to expect.
- Encourage members not to feel compelled to share or do anything until they are feeling ready.

- Enforce rules about speaking in a respectful ways toward others.
- Check in with each group member regularly to help frame and understand how the group events are being perceived and incorporated.
- Get permission from individuals before intervening.
- Encourage the group members to be supportive with one another.
- Emphasize the importance of confidentiality.
- Have a set of ground rules that are enforced consistently.
- Model ways to handle interpersonal conflict so it can be seen as productive and not something to be avoided.
- Interventions should be intentional, based on individuals and the stage of group process.

## BASIC PARAMETERS FOR GROUP

It is important to tailor the group parameters around space, time one has available, and goals for the group. It is critical that the physical space is large enough to encourage interaction and is private in terms of soundproofing and confidentiality. For each member to get enough engagement and contact, I have found that the optimal group size is between eight and 12 members. The time range of 1½ to 2 hours seems to work well for individuals to interact in this format.

The number of sessions is best connected to the goals one has for the experience. An 8- or 12-week short-term format might work best at the start if there is a specific behavioral focus, such as learning healthy ways of coping with unemployment, preparing to be a new father, or dealing with divorce/separation. Rotating short-term groups has the advantage of more focus, especially if there is a skill-based curriculum. Process-oriented groups, which involve exploring intergroup relationships and sharing long-term psychological patterns, tend to take longer to develop trust and might function better in a longer format. Extended weekend groups or 1-week formats might work best if there is access to a retreat setting that might allow for concentrated meeting time with individuals who will be together only for that period of time (Englar-Carlson & Stevens, 2014).

The leader should decide ahead of time whether the group is open or closed. An open group allows members to come and go and tends to have the basic goal of being a place to talk about personal issues with a qualified therapist or group leader. Members may have lower levels of trust because a new person might appear in the group on any given week. A group for homeless residents or a group for people who come for addiction treatment to a therapeutic facility, where the membership varies based on admittance into the program, are good open group examples. A closed group requires members to commit to attending and doesn't accept new members once the group has started. This tends to nurture more intimate interpersonal relationships because of ongoing sharing and increasing disclosures.

## QUALITIES OF EFFECTIVE GROUP THERAPISTS

Effective group leaders are characterized by their vision, compassion, willingness to respond, inherent valuing of members, team orientation, and ability to teach new skills (Kottler & Englar-Carlson, 2014). Group leaders need to attend to not only each individual in the group but also the group process as a whole. If a group is more psychoeducational, then the leader needs to prepare materials for presentations, questions for members, and exercises for application. This type of group has the advantages of focusing on a particular topic and encouraging discussion. The disadvantage is that the group members tend to depend on the leader for structure and are less likely to generate their own material in the group sessions.

In a therapeutic process group, characterized by members bringing in material from their own lives to discuss in the group context, leaders must stay attuned to each member's personal issues, encourage sharing through active listening, and model and teach effective communication skills. Active listening and interventions such as reflecting, interpreting, reframing, confronting, summarizing, and questioning are at the core of group facilitation (Kottler & Englar-Carlson, 2014). Group therapists must also "direct the traffic" of communication within the group by knowing when to challenge members who may be avoiding conflict, to make connections between member disclosures that might not initially seem relevant, to encourage links between members who seem to be talking just to the leader, and to support individuals who have taken self-disclosure risks to which the group has not responded.

It is also important for therapists to be aware of the range of behavior that each individual might likely use in the group setting and to supportively challenge them to stretch their skill set. For instance, quieter group members might count on the therapist noticing and calling on them for their input. By compassionately identifying this dynamic as a pattern, the therapist might ask an individual to "see what it would be like" to be more assertive in the group.

Adding a group coleader allows a second set of eyes to be on the individuals who are not the center of attention at the moment. Subtle nonverbal cues can give the group coleaders feedback about how others are feeling or experiencing the content and process. Although one therapist might encourage an individual member to share, the other might notice tears welling up in an observing member's eyes and be able to turn the attention back to the reactor and what he or she might be experiencing.

In process-oriented groups, leaders address elements that affect the group as a whole. Rather than just respond to an individual, the therapist can address the entire group with an observation of the process. Systems theory suggests that all groups of people, from families to organizations, tend to organize themselves into predictable patterns like forming subgroups and alliances between individuals and developing social norms and subtle rules about communication to preserve homeostasis (Connors & Caple, 2005). By noticing when the group is discussing an emotionally difficult topic or if there is an impasse in communication, the facilitator can add insight about group as a system. Process dynamics might include who is communicating with whom and how, which members seems to more supportive of one another, how conflicts are being resolved, or what roles members are playing in dictating the direction of the group. Sometimes nonverbal cues such as a lack of eye contact when speaking to certain individuals, arm crossing or fidgeting while someone speaks, or silence following a member's verbalizations may be significant indicators of potential confusion about the group's directions, distrust of certain members, impatience with how someone is communicating, or dissatisfaction with the nature of the group interactions and need to be addressed holistically.

## GROUP STAGES

Although no two therapy groups are identical, they do move through a common set of stages that reflect the developmental nature of how individuals connect and coalesce. On the basis of observation and research, the early, middle, and late phases of the group process have been described by several authors in unique ways (see Corey, 2016; Day, 2007; Kottler & Englar-Carlson, 2014; Yalom & Leszcz, 2005).

### Early Stage

Early group development is often characterized by a testing of the waters in terms of trust and inclusion. Members search for commonality, safety, and a sense that they can relate to the others in the group. Although initially cautious and deferential to the group leader, who must model and teach how to be in the group, the communication in the early stages of the group often seems channeled toward finding common ground. Unless there is a participant who shares too much too fast, the group members will incrementally reveal information in a way that is tolerable to the group and stirs the least amount of anxiety. Anxiety tolerance will increase in the group as the least revealing member expresses more than he or she has previously. Once the group has found common footing in terms of level of disclosure and comfort in the predictability of the group, the group will naturally move toward topics that are less safe.

### Middle Stage

The middle stage is characterized by members' willingness to discuss issues that may not fit with previously established norms for disclosure. Because there is a basic trust level, there is less need to discuss concerns that are related to inclusion and belonging. Instead, the group can handle discussing differences of opinion and perception about goals, the nature of relationships, and past shame-laden behavior that has brought the individual to group. This may also include questioning the leader, awareness of contradictions in what others are sharing, and a willingness to disagree and engage in conflict. In process groups, this phase may also involve the sharing of emotions like anger, frustration, and sadness, which are often held back in the early development of the group.

The middle stage is often seen as exciting, productive, and engaging to members (Kottler & Englar-Carlson, 2014). By learning to work through conflict, members are more willing to give honest feedback and self-disclose in ways they previously believed were too risky in a group of people they didn't know well. By allowing for differences, group members can learn from one another in a way that adds to their understanding of self and others. With guidance from the leader, individuals can see how they might project their own experiences and emotional states onto others. This gives members a new way to learn about aspects of themselves that might have previously been hidden. It also makes interpersonal feedback more productive because it involves taking in both how others perceive you and how you might be seeing others through your personal lens. Often the group feels as if its members are learning and growing psychologically, which marks the group identity as productive and not risk averse rather than just a safe space. The test for members at this stage is to not be overwhelmed by new information, as old defenses are being regularly challenged and may not work as well as they did prior to the experience. The new ways may take time to absorb and integrate. For instance, an individual who always saw himself as cynical about his ability to express positive emotions might find that he now regularly smiles and laughs in the group. This seems like a positive outcome, but he has very little experience of himself as happy, so it may feel strange to him.

In the later middle stage of group, integration of new ways of thinking and acting becomes more normalized. The group is seen as a place to explore, take risks, and test out new learning. Often group members feel connected in ways they rarely do in their regular lives, almost as if the group takes on the feel of a family. Many family of origin issues may manifest themselves more productively in this stage. Rather than being intrusive, these issues provide insight into how one was raised and what one considers normal and can be a springboard to making choices about acting differently in the present.

## Final Stage

In the final stage, group members are aware of the experience coming to an end. Depending on the length of the group, it is important for the therapist to encourage members to share what they got from their time in the group. Often this involves talking about changes that have occurred, giving feedback to group members about their progress, and usually acknowledging which individuals were significant to their growth. In this stage, there also might be increased anxiety about the group ending, because it has provided a safe and challenging space for psychological growth. By acknowledging the ending, the group members may also be triggered by other loss experiences in their lives. It is not uncommon for there to be less deep sharing as group members begin to divest some of their commitment to the group process. Hopefully the group therapist can facilitate productive discussions about the process of loss, finding meaning in an experience that is coming to an end and taking the learning into the world outside the group.

Groups are powerful vehicles for intra- and interpersonal growth. Benefits include getting feedback on one's interpersonal style, learning new ways of interacting, and gaining a more universal perspective on one's own life. Early in the life of a group, leaders need to create conditions that encourage safety and trust. In the middle stage, they should provide challenge and encouragement, and in the final stage they should help members deal with loss by finding meaning in their learning and its application in their lives.

# 4

# Making Group Psychotherapy Work for Men

Many benefits result from combining the Deepening approach with group therapy for men. As mentioned in Chapter 3, group psychotherapy expands what can be experienced and learned beyond the one-to-one relationship of individual work. This chapter highlights how to make the group male friendly, the types of themes men discuss in group, the stages typically found in a process-oriented men's group, and how the Deepening conflict zones emerge in the men's group setting. Part III of the book will take you inside a process-oriented men's group in an intimate way, allowing you to see many of the principles, introduced here, in action.

## CREATING A MALE-FRIENDLY GROUP THERAPY ENVIRONMENT

It is important to anticipate the potential issues that might stymie a group of men meeting to discuss their inner lives. By first meeting with each man individually, the group leader can explain the purpose and process of the group, reducing the ambiguity and in turn lowering some of the initial anxiety. This initial discussion also gives each man an opportunity to share some of his fears and anticipation. These feelings can then be addressed in a positive and supportive way by the therapist. If the group is to have a focus or theme, such as dealing with depression, coping with loss, handling divorce, or managing anger, it is essential that group members understand the process and limitations.

http://dx.doi.org/10.1037/0000132-005
*Deepening Group Psychotherapy With Men: Stories and Insights for the Journey*,
by F. E. Rabinowitz

Unlike a mixed-gender group, the men's group must address the unfamiliar dynamics of men talking about personal issues without the buffer or facilitation of women (unless the group includes a woman coleader; see Chapter 12 for more about this). The group leader can anticipate these issues by normalizing the discomfort and using it as a springboard for discussion in the group. Early sessions may need more structure to help the men get a running start in their conversations. The group leader might also be more self-disclosing than in individual therapy so that the men in the group can see him as someone who has also been working on his issues. By sharing some of his struggles as a man, including relationship challenges or other obstacles he has overcome, a male group leader might become more genuine, less perfect, and less authoritative in the eyes of the members. This encourages more identification and engenders trust that the group facilitator will not be judging a man for not living up to a fantasized masculine ideal. A female group leader will also be expected to self-disclose but will need to demonstrate through her empathy and nonjudgmental comments that men in the group can be open and forthcoming about a wide range of topics (Sweet, 2012).

By talking early about the cultural norms of masculinity, the men can usually find some common ground around expectations they may have had to live up to. In some groups, showing clips from films such as *Glengarry Glen Ross, Braveheart, Sideways, The Shawshank Redemption, Fight Club,* or *About Schmidt* might encourage a deeper conversation about what it means to be a man (Rabinowitz, 2014b).

Because many men have been more socialized to be more "doing" oriented, I have introduced physical activities such as molding clay, drawing, stretching, pushing against each other, hitting a punching bag, or smashing a tennis racquet on a pillow as a way to share frustration, anger, sadness, or emotions not easily verbalized (Rabinowitz & Cochran, 2002). Not only do these actions often lead to a deeper expression of what a man is feeling, they also tend to open up the discussion among members about their fears of being emotionally vulnerable and more fully expressive.

## THEMES OF A MEN'S GROUP

Almost anything can be brought up in a men's group. Although a men's group may focus on a specific aspect of masculinity or a psychological issue such as anger management or trauma recovery, there are questions and themes that seem to reoccur when men are brought together in this environment (Rabinowitz, 2014a).

- What does it mean to be a man?
- How did your family of origin impact you as a man?
- What strategies did you learn in your family about how to handle problems?
- What significant events or traumas have impacted you in your life?
- What does it take for you to trust other men with your vulnerability?

- How have you handled betrayals and disappointments in your life?
- What are some of your secrets that you have been hesitant to share with other men?
- What significance does shame and self-judgment have in your life?
- What is the nature of your relationship with your father? Your mother? Your siblings? How has that impacted you in your role as a man, father, worker, partner?
- How do you feel about your role as worker?
- What is the nature of power and control, and where do you feel its impact in your life?
- What is love, and how do you express it? What keeps you from loving?
- What have you learned about sexuality in your life?
- How do you experience others' sexuality that might be different from yours?
- How have you dealt with anxiety, depression, and fear?
- How do you handle your more primitive impulses?
- How do you deal with your physical self, including aging, injury, and illness?
- How can you expand your emotional repertoire?
- What are your struggles with addictions?
- What does it mean to have a "dark side"?
- What are your goals, fantasies, and expectations for the future?
- What is your passion? How do you reignite this in your life?
- What is the nature of your intimate relationships, and what might you do to improve communication?
- How can you build a psychologically healthy life?
- What can I learn from the relationships I am developing in the group?
- How can ancient myths and stories be applied to your life?
- What are your creative outlets for emotional expression?
- What have you lost? What is unfinished? How do you handle losses in your life?

## STAGES OF MEN'S THERAPY GROUPS

### Building Trust

Entering the men's group parallels the male journey from the safety of the mother's orbit as a little boy into the world of men. Like a spaceship entering the earth's atmosphere, defenses are on high alert to avoid being consumed by the potential shaming inherent in traditional masculinity. The vulnerability it takes to explore oneself in a group of men does not come easily. Often a positive individual therapy experience opens a man up for the possibility of sharing more within the group setting. Therapists who lead men's groups have to be sensitive to the violation of the typical male social norms that the group process requires of its members. By anticipating the conflict zones activated by the group setting, the leader of the men's group can better structure and intervene in a way to deepen the experience for the members.

The early stage of the group is built around creating trust. Like the groups described in Chapter 3, men must establish some common ground with one another before they can move deeper into discussing personal issues. I have found that group members are more likely to share more extensively when given specific directions, especially at the start of a group. For instance, the men might be asked to introduce themselves by name, profession, and where they grew up geographically (fairly low-risk disclosures) but also to share an aspect of their life that might not be so obvious to an outsider. This "ante up" of a difficult disclosure is a risk that has benefits in terms of bonding (Rabinowitz, 2014b) and often leads to finding personal commonalities that exceed typical starting male conversations. The more revealing the disclosures, the greater the chance that the others in the group will loosen their restrictions on what they will say in the group. The group leader might continue to bring up a topic or question each session in the early stage to give the men a familiar way to enter the conversation. By finding commonalities around the rules of masculinity, difficulties with expressing emotions other than anger, and struggles in relationships, for instance, men in the group begin to bond around the idea that they are not alone in their private thoughts and feelings.

## Deepening the Connection

As the men in the group begin to recognize their common connections around many of the themes of their lives, the leader may need to do less prompting for discussion. In my experience, the men will begin to spontaneously discuss conflicts in their current lives and to reflect on what had been discussed in previous sessions, including reacting to what other men have shared in the group. Often a man will explore areas of his life that he had not previously revealed to anyone outside an individual therapist. This increased vulnerability is often accompanied by more willingness for the men in the group to engage with the emotional level of sharing. Members are more willing to give honest feedback about how they perceive another's revelations. The men's group is unique because this kind of conversation has rarely been modeled, so there is trepidation about how much to share. The leader is often needed to help with encouragement and to model how to talk about experiences that include not just a description but also the emotions that are felt. This is almost like a new level of language that is shared. The use of metaphors and analogies allows men to feel comfortable sharing the experience in a rich and engaging manner (McKelley, 2014). The other quality of this stage of the group is that conflict can be approached and is productive. Because trust has been established, it is easier for men to disagree and stay connected in the process. In the trust-building stage, conflict is threatening and often means that a man might not be accepted if he disagrees or has a negative reaction to another member. In this stage, each man can share where he is coming from with less defensiveness, knowing that he is accepted and trusted even when there are disagreements.

### Integrating Learning

In this stage of the group, there is sufficient belief in the process of sharing, that it is possible to bring this openness into relationships outside of the group room. Men report that they are more open to significant others and willing to face conflict in their relationships. Inside the group, there is an enhanced sense of support for each man's desires, wishes, and dreams. The group is an encouraging place to share how each man wants to better his life. Changing life patterns is not easy, but with the support of a group of men who are trusted, it can be approached. The men know one another well enough to be supportive of each person's individual goals. Whereas for one man it might be having the courage to go out on dates, for another it might be having the guts to leave an unhealthy relationship.

### Letting Go

The last stage of the group is characterized by an acknowledgment of the support, feedback, and genuineness that each man has brought to the group experience. If the group is time limited, the last sessions are often devoted to reviewing progress and encouraging the men to continue to pursue their personal goals beyond the life of the group. This can be a fairly emotional time, when the group members realize how much they have come to rely on the group for support. Some group members may start to emotionally distance themselves as the group comes to a close. Group leaders can point out the withdrawal and connect it to the impending loss of the group experience and the relationships that have developed.

## THE DEEPENING CONFLICT ZONES IN THE GROUP SETTING

### The Dependency Conflict

If there is one masculine norm that crosses cultures, it is the importance of not being dependent on anyone or anything. As reviewed earlier, the dependency conflict for men seems to have its origins in childhood and is then reinforced throughout life with the traditional male code. Men are supposed to be strong and autonomous. Dependency sounds like weakness. As young boys we were dependent on our parents and caregivers, but as men we expect to make our own decisions.

The group situation brings men together in a way that activates some of these dependency concerns. Not only is the group facilitator given the power to lead, but the demand in the group is to be honest in sharing. Both of these create a dynamic that can make a man feel as if he must rely on the leader for structure and safety and must trust the other men not to take advantage of his revealing his inner world. This situation leads to a feeling of not being fully in control of how the group dynamic will proceed. In my 35 years of leading groups, I have found that men in the group simultaneously experience this dynamic of vulnerability and initially respond with their typical defenses, including staying superficial, minimizing emotion, exaggerating the narrative, being silent, or rationalizing their experiences as "no big deal."

Although in many group situations men rely on the women present to facilitate the interpersonal realm, the men's group takes away this dynamic (Brooks, 1996). Men are left to themselves to interact without this familiar factor. Although dependency on women in interpersonal relationships seems normative, the absence of women group members creates even more dependency on the leader to manage the emotional needs of the group.

In individual therapy, trust builds in the relationship with the therapist on the basis of repeated exposure to supportive interventions rather than threatening ones. Eventually a male client will begin to lower his walls, share his inner thoughts and feelings more readily, and be able to notice when he is not being open. In the group setting, even if the therapist is trusted to not take advantage of his vulnerability, the group member is now faced with men he doesn't know. Despite the intellectual framing that is done by the facilitator around mutual vulnerability in the group and the benefits of group therapy, many men do not respond initially with openness (Brooks, 1998a). It is more likely that they will employ typical strategies for safety, which may include shows of psychological strength, minimal verbal expression, and intellectual distancing from vulnerable emotions.

The following techniques facilitate issues related to ambivalence about relational dependency in the group:

- Recall childhood scenes when one felt scared or worried.
- Prompt discussions about the nature of one's relationships with other boys or men.
- Share a longing or wish about a significant relationship in one's life (e.g., mother, father, caretaker).
- Direct group members to ask directly for support from another member following a vulnerable disclosure.

## Managing Grief and Loss Experiences

By being encouraged to tell the stories that make up their life experiences, the men in the group often share painful, joyful, and poignant recollections. The men act as witnesses to one another and provide a container for the emotional intensity inherent in deeper sharing. When the group is functioning well, stories about loss often arise, as this is a common pathway to deeper emotions for many men (Rabinowitz & Cochran, 2002). By mutually sharing difficult, emotional material, the group becomes a safe space to air internal conflict, including grief and sadness. It is not uncommon for one man to take a risk to share feelings of loss, which then elicits permission for others to do the same. Although initially reluctant to go too deep, the intimacy created in the group changes the traditional male norms around emotional self-expression. Everyone in the group can relate to loss experiences. When the sharing of losses is treated with dignity, care, and desire to understand what a man has gone through, the group becomes a safer place to share difficult emotions (Cochran & Rabinowitz, 1996; Rabinowitz & Cochran, 2002). In the outside world, it is easy to dismiss one's losses with statements like "No one wants to hear me whine about something that happened a long time ago" or "Everyone goes through this. No big deal." Men display support with one another through verbal and nonverbal actions. Verbally, men are encouraged to share their reactions and find it natural to have empathy for the individual who tells his story of loss. Nonverbally, it is not uncommon for men to use eye contact or a caring touch or embrace as a way to show support to a man who has shared some of his pain (Rabinowitz, 1991).

The following techniques facilitate issues related to loss and grief in the group:

- Use guided imagery to recall a significant loss experienced as a boy or man.
- Prompt a discussion about what makes you sad.
- Ask men to bring in a picture of someone they have lost and talk about it to the group.
- Spend time focusing on body awareness as one speaks about a loss.
- Encourage a gestalt empty chair dialogue with someone who has been lost, or have another member play the part in a psychodrama.

### Challenging Masculine Self-Structures in the Group Setting

For many men, the initial reaction to being in a group of men is to compete for leadership through storytelling and displays of masculine strength. This might take the form of talking about his job or what neighborhood he lives in. Defining oneself through traditional masculine norms is often what men have been socialized to do. The men's group flips this dynamic. Instead of being rewarded for showing how strong, accomplished, or great one can be, the men are reinforced for displaying the authentic emotions that accompany their experience. Over time, the man who hides behind his bravado mask in the group will be challenged to be more forthcoming with the emotions that lie under his defense system. Challenge does not mean shaming. Most men will have empathy for the traditional defenses that accompany difficult emotions. The group helps by being interested in the story. The group members can acknowledge the strength of the man while asking him to be more specific with the emotions he is feeling as he shares. Those who struggle can be aided by self-disclosures from individuals who can share what they felt. This not only models the safe expression of emotion but also shows a depth of understanding that many men are not used to encountering.

The following techniques facilitate issues related to confronting masculine self-structures in group:

- Encourage men to exaggerate the expectations they feel about being a man.

- Discuss the rules of masculinity and how each man feels about those values.
- Ask a man to dialogue with the perceived enforcer of the masculine rules.
- Share one's shame at not living up to some inner expectations, usually connected to a male authority or father figure.

### Doing Versus Being

Often, many of the men in the group want to problem solve one another's issues. Men in Western culture tend toward a "doing" orientation when faced with a dilemma (Winnicott, 1988). Although it is a positive trait to be a good problem solver in the material world, it is often a mistake to override the feeling element when trying to understand the emotions that accompany a painful human situation. Men have been taught to try to fix something that is wrong, but if one doesn't fully comprehend the depth or complexity of an emotional problem, it can be premature and miss the point. The leader in the men's group setting often has to remind group members to stay with an emotion or reaction before moving in the direction of solving. Men will give advice, share their experiences, but often don't take the time to stay with a feeling. Exercises that encourage awareness of the body and increased attention to the emotional elements of a problem can help men be less intellectual and more in touch with how it is impacting them. Over time, group members will often call out one another on the problem-solving mode and catch themselves. It is often a source of humor when it becomes obvious that everyone in the room has fallen into the socialized behavior to fix whatever problems someone has shared.

The following techniques facilitate issues related to doing and being in group:

- Rather than talk about a feeling, have a man act it out by striking pillows or hitting a punching bag to get at deeper emotions.
- Ask a man to stay with the feelings in his body rather than explain them away intellectually.
- Have men in the group physically hold back a member from moving toward someone or something he wants to get him to actively engage his body in the emotion.
- Discuss the differences between trying to actively solve a problem and taking time to "be" with the problem before acting on it.

## EXPOSING THE WOUNDS AS A PORTAL TO DEPTH

Ultimately, the group will deepen as the men expose their emotional wounds. The shared exposure makes almost nothing taboo for the group discussion. By sharing the details and circumstances of the wounding, each man opens the portals to emotional depth that lie at his core. The witnessing by others in the group highlights its significance and gives the man a new lived experience that can help him be more open about who he is. Typically, this level of openness does not occur right away. It takes time to let each man reveal himself in tolerable doses. In my experience as a group leader, when a man shares too much too fast, he will have a "shame rebound." This reaction often occurs following the group session, and if not addressed it may be enough for a man to drop out of the group. The group leader must push men to share more while not overwhelming their defenses. Sometimes a man who is in immediate pain will bring this raw level of intensity into the group. Although he may get support through the crisis, it will take time for him to integrate it into a more in-depth understanding of its meaning. Many of the members will share parts of their story initially and gauge the trust level of the group. This incremental sharing allows for the individual's defenses to keep up with the potential shame that might be elicited if information is revealed too quickly. The shared wounds typically center around feelings of abandonment by significant others in one's life; the betrayal of trust by someone who had been emotionally close; or trauma from an injury, accident, or death. These wounds are often accompanied by shame, as the private self feels inherently defective or flawed (Kaufman, 1992).

For some men, the only open channel is anger. Feeling frustrated is a general state that often has not been titrated into more complex emotional states. By allowing anger to arise in the group, a man might find a channel to other emotions. It is not uncommon for a man to be encouraged to use the tennis racquet to hit pillows or to punch the bag as a way to get to the sadness, jealousy, fear, or hurt that might lie beneath the anger and frustration. Sometimes an interpersonal conflict will arise in the group that has been triggered by one group member's sharing. By encouraging members to respond with their own honest feelings, men learn how to work through difficult emotions in the group setting. A man might not like how another member is talking about a relationship, work, or family. This feeling can be an opening to discover what wound portal has been triggered and to do some emotional work around it. By allowing for the projection of feeling into another man's story, men can use the interpersonal environment to re-own that which they see in the other. In challenging the male norms about sharing vulnerable emotions, men learn to feel more comfortable sharing authentically with one another inside and outside the group.

The following techniques facilitate issues related to exposing the wound as a portal to depth in the group:

- Lead a discussion on wounds and traumas that men have had in their lives.
- Ask men to share where in their bodies some of their wounds reside.
- Use physical exercises like striking pillows or hitting a punching bag to tap emotion that accompanies an emotional wound.
- Encourage the group to give feedback when a man shares pain both verbally and physically.

Whereas a men's therapy group has many of the qualities of a mixed-gender process group, the men's group leader must face some unique and challenging dynamics. The biggest obstacle is running into the socialized tendency for men to be cautious about sharing their vulnerability with other men. With preparation and initial structure by the therapist, most men will find sharing their inner experience in the group to be relieving and healing rather than shame inducing. The later stages of a men's group are characterized by more expressivity, willingness to work through interpersonal conflict, and an integration of learning from the group interactions. The Deepening conflict zones do manifest in the men's group and can be addressed through structured interventions.

# II

# STORIES MEN BRING TO GROUP THERAPY

## INTRODUCTION: STORIES MEN BRING TO GROUP THERAPY

To give you, the reader, a sense of the variations of the Deepening therapy process, I introduce in Part II 10 men who exemplify a cross-section of the types of men a clinician might engage in treatment. They do not represent the full gamut of men, nor are they so severely psychologically disturbed that psychotherapy might not be effective. As noted earlier, each story corresponds to that of a real person that I invited to be part of the men's therapy group, but my portrayals here alter many details to protect their privacy. I have tried to be as honest as possible in giving a sense of my personal reactions, therapeutic concerns, and analysis of the process. At the end of each therapy story, I ask the reader to reflect on what has transpired in terms of your own experience, the most significant issues raised, and how you might respond if you were working with the client. I also share my thoughts about why the individual might be a good fit in the men's group and what the potential challenges might be.

In each of the following 10 stories, I take you through an unfolding process between me as the therapist and my client, as I interact with him. This is the Deepening process, which you will see elaborated in a group setting in Part III. During individual therapy, each man in his own way will initially resist the connection between us. He will take measures to protect himself from the shame he experiences in relation to the discomfort he faces. But, eventually, each individual will take the risk to trust me to be the receiver of his inner battle. He will confront the consequences of having not known how to handle difficult situations in his life. Through my nonjudgmental presence, I will encourage him to embrace a fresh and compassionate relationship with himself. By accepting uncertainty and some degree of discomfort, each man will test out new ways of being in the world that feel more congruent and genuine for him.

As you get to know each man profiled in Part II, I invite you to envision the men with whom you work in your therapy practice. What are their strengths? What could each one contribute in a group situation? What could they learn from each other in a group setting?

# 5

# Excavating the Dark Passages

Although we see others mainly from the outside for the roles they play, a rich interior exists, usually out of sight. In my role as psychotherapist, I am given permission to help shine the light on some of the dark passages of a man's inner world. Often a man will try to hide these elements from others but pay the price with emotional turmoil. In this chapter we meet two men who are duty bound by their work and the way they try to live their lives. Kevin, a police officer, does his best to be an honest, ethical public servant but is frustrated by the lack of support from colleagues and is hurt deeply by betrayal in his personal life. Tony, a successful business owner and man of faith, lives with inner trepidation about the secrets he has kept from those important to him. Both use the therapy process to work through the conflicts between the moral and more emotional aspects of themselves.

## KEVIN: THE ANGRY COP

"This is stupid. I don't need to be here, so let's cut to the chase, Doc. The idiots in my department act like it is all on me. Fuck them!"

These were the first words out of Kevin's mouth in our very first session. I was wondering why I agreed to take this client on, given how busy I was. It is hard enough to do good therapy. When a man is coming in against his will, it is almost impossible to make progress.

http://dx.doi.org/10.1037/0000132-006
*Deepening Group Psychotherapy With Men: Stories and Insights for the Journey,*
by F. E. Rabinowitz

The fire of anger is a great defense because it pushes people away. Most of the time, anger clears a path for the individual and isolates him from those who are close. Sometimes alcohol or drugs exacerbate and loosen the inhibition on its expression. People start to steer clear of the angry person's wake, and in the end he has no challenges to his personhood. The problem is that the isolation does not actually help the individual mature or grow, and if he runs into someone else who is triggered, there is bound to be a conflict. Often the only chance for therapeutic success is to get at what is underneath the frustration and rage.

### In Trouble Again

Kevin, a 33-year-old White police officer, was told he needed to "clean up his act" or risk being permanently fired from his job as a detective. He was on leave for having gotten into a fistfight with one of his colleagues when they were out at a bar after a shift. Witnesses reported that Kevin had escalated an argument, which turned physical. Kevin had stitches across his left eyebrow, his left eye was swollen shut, and his nose was crooked and bruised. He looked like a prizefighter who had gone 10 rounds. Kevin chose to see me because of my specialization in working with men. I have to admit that fighting has never been my solution to conflict. If anything, I have avoided fights my whole life. Rather than fight, I always worked hard to understand where the other person was coming from. This usually deescalated conflict, even if I might have been justified in my anger. I have had to learn to "own" my anger. Often I have been too quick to reconcile or see the other person's point of view. Obviously, this helps me as a therapist. I can stay calm while my client vents, but it hinders me in having a grasp of someone who might strike first and think later.

"Kevin, I'm not making assumptions. I want to hear your take on things. My job is to understand and help if I can," I responded.

"You know, you are not the first shrink I've seen. I've had to see counselors since I was a kid. I guess it hasn't done me much good."

"What do you mean by that?" I asked, reacting a bit to Kevin's confrontational style.

"Well. Here I am sitting in your psychologist office, once again in trouble for fighting. Pretty lame. You'd think I would learn that this is what happens when you lose it."

"What do you think keeps you from learning the lesson?" I asked.

"Good shrink question. I think I have been asked this about a hundred times in my life. I get pissed off and something snaps. The next thing I know I'm yelling, and in some extreme cases in a physical altercation, as we say in law enforcement."

"Can we talk some about this particular situation? It seems pretty serious, given the possibility of you losing your job."

"What do you want to know? Specifics? I have been in the police department for the past 11 years. Worked my way up from beat cop to detective. I am not just saying this, but I've been one of the most productive officers this department has had. My arrest and conviction record has been pretty stellar. I think they want to keep me, but I've also ruffled enough feathers that maybe that is not so true anymore."

"What do you mean 'ruffled enough feathers'?" I asked.

"Well, you know, the politics. I am pretty straight-edged. I don't do drugs. Even that night in the bar, I had just one beer. It wasn't alcohol-infused rage. But some of the other detectives are less than clean in their personal lives. I think I threaten them because I play by the rules. The guy I fought is an ass. He thinks he's hot shit. He started bragging about some drug bust he made, and I know he lucked out. He was off duty and happened to run into this big dealer at a rock concert, who tried to sell him something. I had been tracking that guy for over a year. So anyway, he made the bust and then started trashing my investigation to the other guys in the bar. I told him to shove it. He's trained in mixed martial arts and had a few beers in him. The next thing I know, we are going at it."

"Sounds like you felt he had it coming."

"Damn right. But I am the one here. He's probably off on some Hawaiian vacation with one of his many girlfriends."

"You seem envious." My intuition was that Kevin felt as if he was being punished for playing by the rules and that others seemed to get rewarded for their less-than-stand-up behavior.

"Of course. He hasn't had to work that hard. I have busted my ass and overcome a ton of shit. Now it could all get thrown away because of him."

### Entering His World

As I listened to Kevin, I was drawn to his story. He was sharing more than I expected. I wanted to know more, but I was also cognizant of letting him reveal to me at his own pace. I wondered whether previous therapists had tried to calm Kevin down rather than try to understand his anger. By listening and understanding his reaction, it felt as if I had earned some of his trust. Kevin showed less agitation and was more verbally articulate than I had expected in a first session. We agreed on weekly meetings for the next 8 weeks, which the department was paying for. I let him know that I was his therapist and that I would keep confidentiality (unless he was dangerous to himself or others). They had a psychologist who would assess him for his job once he had completed his counseling. I made it clear that I wanted to help him work on finding ways to better express himself so that anger wasn't his only outlet.

### Naming His Strength

In our next session, Kevin was a bit less wound-up. He was dressed casually in a T-shirt and sweats. His 6-foot 2-inch build was muscular. He had a few days of stubble. I picked up where we left off in our first session.

"Kevin, you had mentioned that you had been seeing counselors since childhood. Can you tell me what it was like for you growing up?"

Kevin hesitated and took a deep breath.

"Not a pretty picture. I am guessing you figured that out already if you are as good a psychologist as I think you might be."

"What do you mean?" I asked. Kevin seemed to set me up with a teaser before he was willing to talk about his personal life. My active interest in his story seemed to let him know it was okay to reveal more.

"I grew up in a very rough area in L.A. Dad left when I was a baby; raised by a mom who didn't seem to care much. Not a good combination," he stated with very little emotion. This wasn't hard for him to share. I could tell he had told this story before. This was the CliffsNotes version. I would need to know more.

Over the course of our meeting, Kevin gave me a more in-depth rundown of his experiences as an only child, growing up in poverty. He was constantly in trouble at school for truancy and fighting, yet school was the safest place he knew. He recalled teachers who had taken him under their wings and supported his intellectual development.

"I got beat up every single day of my life from first grade to eighth grade." As a nonfighter, I was incredulous. How could a kid go through this every day of his life at that age or at any age?

"That must have been horrible for you." I tried to empathize.

"You know, I don't see it that way. The neighborhood bullies just saw me as something to play with. It was pretty predictable."

"Still. You must have been scared to go to school."

"You are probably figuring this out about me. I am a tough motherfucker. I realized that if you are hit enough, physical pain loses its power. It was like a part of my day. After a while it just doesn't hurt. I actually looked forward to the adventure of going to school. It was a jungle fight. Got my adrenaline going. I felt like I earned my place in school."

Wow. I had never heard anyone tell me a story like that. Because I avoided getting hit my whole life, Kevin's nonchalant experience with physical abuse was foreign. I could hardly imagine having the crap beat out of me and then live to tell the story without being traumatized. On the other hand, I think Kevin just developed a high threshold for pain. It also dawned on me that getting in fights might be something so familiar to him that he actually was pretty clueless about why everyone was so upset by it. I was also reminded that each individual interprets his experience uniquely and that just because Kevin was assaulted, it does not mean that I should assume he was damaged from this. In fact, as Kevin went on, I sensed he gained strength from his ability to take punishment and not give up.

"So you got beat up every day through eighth grade and then it stopped? What happened after that?"

"I ended up becoming part of a gang where we had each other's backs. In fact, one of the kids who used to beat me up became one of my protectors in high school. It was like a club, family. No one messed with us in high school. I took martial arts classes after school and really learned to be more efficient and skilled in my ability to defend myself."

"I can tell you are a super intelligent man. You said that some of your teachers mentored you?" I replied.

"Yes. I was fortunate. Even though we didn't have any books or even a TV at home, my teachers in middle school and high school gave me stuff to read. I ate it up. I read *Lord of the Flies, Animal Farm, 1984, A Tale of Two Cities, Call of the Wild, Treasure Island, Moby-Dick, Heart of Darkness.* This stuff really informed me about my experience. It provided a narrative. I think I ended up reading all of Shakespeare's works in my senior year of high school. My English teacher was an aficionado."

Kevin was blowing my mind. Here I thought I was going to be dealing with a rogue cop who might have limited insight about his predicament. Instead I was in the presence of an extraordinary human being who not only had survived a harsh childhood but had made the most of it. He did have his rough edges, but there was way more to work with than I had imagined.

"So you are telling me that books saved your life?" I asked.

"I'm telling you that since I grew up with no parental influences, I was a product of my environment. It was a trip through humanity's most base nature. Reading helped me put context on it. Each of the writers showed me something about how the world worked, and that really saved my life. All the violence, neglect, selfishness, and pettiness made more sense to me. It helped me understand the choices to be made about the kind of person I wanted to be."

"How did you decide to become a police officer?" I asked.

"Well, I ended up getting a scholarship to UCLA and studied English Literature. I didn't quite fit in socially with my peers but made excellent grades in my English classes. I graduated with honors. My professors pushed me to go toward graduate school. I thought about it but decided that I had more to offer doing some public service work. I had been on the wrong end of the law a few times. I admired cops. They were tough but did good work. I liked the thought of combining my impoverished upbringing with my awareness about the human condition. A cop kept order but also had to show compassion for others. That is why it pisses me off when I encounter cops who are just on power trips or who are lazy or who are just pulling a paycheck."

I could sense his anger coming back. He was getting worked up at those who were not giving it their all.

"You seem pissed."

"Fuck, yeah. I lived the shit. I don't have a lot of tolerance for two-faced assholes who say one thing and do another. That fucker Theo who did this to me is pretty rotten. He is disrespectful to women and people of color. He is one of those guys who loves wearing the badge for its power, not for what he is supposed to be doing: protecting people."

"You made a commitment and choice to be a cop. It is hard for you to respect others who don't have that same commitment."

"You know it. That angers me. I don't care what you do, but as long as you are not a hypocrite, I can respect you."

"Sounds like there have been others in your life who have disappointed you." I was thinking that this view of the world came from direct experience.

"I have a whole list of them starting with my dad, my mom, and my ex-wife. Where do you want to start?" I was aware we were near the end of our session, so I summed up our meeting and suggested we start with the betrayal theme next time.

## Finding a Way Forward

I was expecting our third session to start where we left off. Instead Kevin came in angry again. I could see the rage in his eyes. He was wearing a tie and sport coat. His movement into the room was jerky. As he sat down, his cell phone flew out of his pocket onto the floor. Kevin mumbled, reaching to pick up his phone.

"What's going on?" I asked.

"Unbelievable. I just got out of court. My ex-wife's lawyer just took me to the cleaners, and the judge bought it. I am going to have to pay almost half my take-home salary to her. Wow. My attorney told me that there was little chance that would happen, especially since we didn't have kids. She portrayed herself as abused and unable to work, so I will need to pay until she 'gets back on her feet,' which will probably be never."

"Kevin, it's okay. We have some time to talk about this in here. You seem really worked up. Talk to me about your ex-wife. What's her name?"

"Karla. She is a piece of work. Karla is one of the most manipulative bitches I have ever seen. I was such a sucker, and boy am I paying for this one."

"She fooled you? Fill me in on this."

"Another long story."

"We have time."

"I met Karla when I was 29. She was, and is, extremely beautiful, and she knows it. We had a mutual friend who had set us up. I hadn't dated very much and wasn't very experienced with women. Karla had been married when she was very young. Anyway, we hit it off. She seemed very into me, and that blinded me to the things that were screwy with her. Sex was great at the beginning. She was a lot of fun. I was more uptight, and she helped me loosen up. I opened up more to her than anyone in my life. It was a big deal to me."

"Sounds like it started well. What happened?"

"Little to my knowledge, Karla had a bit of an honesty problem, to put it mildly. At first it was little things that I dismissed because I was so into her. Her story about her family was vague and shifting. She originally told me she was an only child, but then later told me she had two stepsisters. When I probed more, she told me that her dad had a second family she only found out about when she was a teenager. She didn't realize that she was engaged to a future detective, so I did some fact checking of my own. Turned out that she actually had two sisters who lived with her. Karla had gotten in trouble with drugs and missing school, and had to leave her family to spend time in juvenile hall. I found this out by talking to her mom."

"So what did you do with this information?"

"I confronted her. She got upset and left for about a week. When she came back, she was very apologetic but she didn't tell me where she went. I got pissed and got a little physical with her, which she used against me."

"Physical?" I was worried about domestic violence and wanted to make sure that I wasn't missing an abuse situation that needed to be reported.

"I was so frustrated, I pushed her against the door. Believe me, if I wanted to hurt her I could have. It was very minor, but she told me that if I ever did that again, she would report it and get me fired from my job as an officer. I backed off, but I distrusted her from that point on. She called the shots in the relationship after that. I just went along. I was afraid she would kill my career."

"Sounds like emotional blackmail."

"Yes. Well, I stupidly let it happen. She went on acting like we were this ideal couple. We ended up getting married. Karla didn't work a regular job. She told me there wasn't anything she was really that interested in. But she was very into shopping and taking good care of herself physically. She always was dressed very sexy and seemed to not be in need of money from me. I worked long hours, so when I got home I was just needing basic stuff, like food, rest, sex, some distracting talk, and watching movies. Karla was good for that, but not much emotional intimacy. I should have been suspicious, but again I convinced myself she was who she said she was. I wished I hadn't found out."

"What do you mean?"

"Karla turned out to be a high-end escort, you know, a prostitute who makes big money from rich johns. I was in shock, but I had her followed when I was at work, and it was true. I found that out about two years ago. Instead of confronting her, I just watched it like I was some kind of voyeur. I felt sorry for myself, and that I was justified in being an asshole to her. I was verbally abusive, not physical. I didn't let on to her that I knew of her secret life. If she pulled the abuse card, I was going to pull the 'you are a whore' card. Inside I was hurt, but that was my own private pain."

True to his nature as a fighter, Kevin had a secret weapon. I believed that he wasn't physically abusive, but he had learned to fight his wife by withholding, acting like he didn't care, and saving the knowledge of her secret life for a grand finale showdown. She was a tough opponent. By not responding to the betrayal, Kevin's anger intensified. His job and home life were worlds where people were dishonest and breaking the rules. In both realms, he was handcuffed by the law, his strong morality, and his own need to win. He was being beat up, maybe even enjoying it in some masochistic way, but he would get his revenge, or so he thought. The court case blew up that scenario. But now I could do my job with him. With his intelligence, ability to reflect, and now willingness to share with me some of what lies beneath the rage, we had a working chance. No easy fixes. This would take some time, but I sensed Kevin was up for it. He had been judged only by his external life, but I would take seriously his internal world.

"So you do feel pain," I said, quite aware of how much he had been beat up in his life.

"Emotional pain hurts worse than physical pain. Betrayal is powerful. I can take a punch, but to get hit with a psychological clusterfuck is harder. Shakespeare wrote Karla's part in Antony and Cleopatra when she betrays Caesar. I should have seen Cleopatra coming."

"The themes Shakespeare wrote keep replaying in your life. I know you are smart and strong, but maybe we can excavate some of that betrayal pain, feel it, understand it, and let it go so you don't carry so much around with you."

"If we can do that, I'll be here every week."

"I'm game. Sounds like I need to brush up on my Shakespeare."

"Don't worry, Doc. I'll keep you on your toes."

## Personal Reflection

- How comfortable are you with anger and its expression? How might you have responded to Kevin's temper and his comments related to physical confrontation in his relationship?
- How do you conceptualize trauma? How do the challenging events that Kevin described in his life impact you personally? How might you have responded in session to his revelations?
- How might Kevin's fears about betrayal play into the therapeutic process? What would be the behavioral cues you might notice if he was feeling disappointment and betrayal in you as a therapist?

## What Makes Kevin a Good Candidate for Group?

Several aspects of Kevin's process encouraged me to consider his becoming a part of the men's group. Although I was impressed by his intelligence and willingness to explore what was going on beneath the surface, it was clear to me that he had very few men in his life with whom he could share his true, authentic self. Kevin's early childhood neglect and abuse and his need to fend for himself left him vulnerable to sensing that potential abandonment or annihilation was imminent. Given what he had been through in terms of work conflict and divorce, I knew that Kevin would benefit from a group of peers who could support him continuing to explore his past relationships and family of origin issues. Although I believed that he might have difficulty with trusting other men, he also had gravitated toward the neighborhood gang as family. He trusted some of his teachers, and he trusted me. I wondered if the vulnerability required to be intimate in the group might be a barrier to his getting close to others. His role as a tough cop protects him in the traditional male world he occupies, but in the men's group he would need to operate outside of that restrictive masculine self-structure. If I could help him through some of his negative projections with guys he didn't know, it might allow him to make the group a place he could experiment with being open and real.

Kevin's portal to his deeper self was through his anger, his main mode of emotional self-expression and his way of protecting himself. I believed that if the group of men assembled could tolerate, and perhaps identify with, his anger, Kevin might get the support he needed. The feedback that Kevin would receive from other men who were also struggling with how to be more expressive and honest with themselves would be invaluable to him. An interpersonally oriented group might provide a safe but challenging laboratory for him to learn about himself in relationships and to get a reality check on how he was perceiving himself and his world.

## TONY: THE SHADOW BEHIND THE GOOD GUY

To be a good man is to be responsible. You will do whatever it takes to uphold your perceived obligations in life. Being a man of duty means a willingness to sacrifice your own needs for those of others. We admire the good guys who do this for family, community, and country. Although extremely admirable, the good guy can also get himself into trouble. Psychiatrist and writer Carl Jung (1983) observed that optimally one should have a balance in one's psyche between self-fulfillment and helping others. When this gets out of balance one way or the other, there are psychological consequences. In the case of the "good guy," it might mean that there is a "shadow" self that starts to operate to compensate for all the conscious self-sacrifice. This might manifest as emotion and behavior that may not be socially acceptable.

As someone who was raised with high morals, I understand the value of being responsible. In Jewish culture, it is called being a mensch. I readily see what is expected of me and try to perform to the best of my ability. I am a master at seeing situations in which my intervention might make a difference. Look anywhere, and someone could use your help. That kid could use some mentoring; that person could use some money; that cause could use some support; that task at work could use some extra focus. After a while, it feels as if being a good guy is really being a fireman who is constantly on call. There is always something I could be helping with, fixing, or contributing to.

I feel very responsible, but I have paid for this. Before engaging in my own psychotherapy, I paid with excessive worry, guilt, and compromises to my physical health. I also found myself wandering into dark places to escape the demands of goodness, like drugs, sex, and extreme risk taking. This knowledge has made me an expert at seeing beyond the good guy persona in men and helping them discover the more shadowy aspects of themselves—passageways that can lead them toward addiction, danger, and frowned-upon social behavior. I have learned that the shadow is a powerful force that cannot be dismissed. Rather, it is in need of channeling toward a creative, passionate outlet to allow it to coexist with the socially responsible self.

## Something Is Not Right

Tony Garcia found me for therapy through a friend. He had never talked to anyone about himself before. Asking for help was not usually in his wheelhouse, but life was feeling "out of control." Tony was a solid, handsome 45-year-old man of Mexican heritage who was complaining of being stressed out by a heavy work schedule and family obligations. I sensed I was in the presence of a "man of duty." He had muscular arms with Christian cross tattoos on his biceps. He also had a large belly that belied some impulsive eating or drinking habits. His brown eyes met mine firmly.

"Doc, something isn't right. I own my own business. I have a great family. I am close to my parents, yet I wake up every morning with a feeling like everything is going to fall apart."

"Say more about that, Tony. What do you mean?" I asked.

"I used to tell myself, don't stress. It will all work out in the end. These days I don't trust that. I just force myself to get up and go through the motions. No one has complained, but I feel like I am not who I used to be."

"Who were you?" I asked.

"You know, confident, strong. Bring on the day. I will give it my all. I was the king of my world. I built a successful business and knew I was better than everyone else."

"And now you can't find that Tony?"

"Exactly. How could he disappear? What happened to me? I feel like I am losing it."

"What does it feel like in your body?" I queried, aware that Tony was most likely experiencing this in a physical way, since his rational self was telling him everything should be fine.

Tony paused to gather his thoughts and find a way to verbalize it. "It's like a big pit of snakes in my chest," he said, pointing to a spot in the middle of his chest above his belly. "I just want it to stop. I went to a cardiologist who ran tests and told me nothing was wrong with me. He said that I needed to learn to control my anxiety. I could use some relief. Can you help me with some techniques to cut down my stress level? I want to feel normal again."

"I hear you. We can work on that, but it would help me if you could first tell me the story of how you got to this point."

Tony looked at me, cleared his throat. "You want to hear the story of my life? I don't think anyone's ever asked me that." I smiled and nodded.

In my experience, most men hold back sharing their personal narrative. When given permission, it is like a lid has been taken off the pressure cooker. Rather than focus on symptoms and diagnosis, I want to hear the story in a man's own words. The unraveling of what is manifesting as stress in the present often has its origins years ago in patterns that make sense only once they are described. It is also a place where a man might give clues to how he is handling the more shadowy elements of his life. Often, however, there is some holding back, especially material that might feel shameful if exposed to a stranger.

## Defined by Responsibility

Tony spent the next 45 minutes telling me his story in his own words. He was the oldest of four children born to immigrant parents from Mexico. Both of his parents worked hard, each with two jobs to make ends meet. As soon as he got home from school, he oversaw his siblings. Tony was a blessing for his parents, who counted on him to make sure his two brothers and sister ate, went to bed, and didn't beat one another up too badly. As he got older, Tony learned to cook, clean, and do whatever he could to take some of the burden off his parents. I commented, "That is a lot to take on at such a young age."

He minimized it. "No choice, Doc. It's what I had to do."

My mind wandered to questions such as, What did this man do as a boy for fun? The shadow finds its outlets through play, and it is really when we lose that sense of playfulness that it finds more deviant manifestations.

In adolescence, Tony began to work with his father on fixing the family car. His dad did all of his own repair work. Tony was a fast learner who quickly became his father's right hand while doing tune-ups and repairs. In fact, Tony ended up getting a job in an auto repair garage when he turned 18. He still lived at home and made sure his paycheck went to some of the family expenses. Tony told me he didn't drink or do drugs, even though he saw other teenagers in his neighborhood indulging. "It was just wrong. I knew it and stayed away from those kids."

Tony made it through school with passing grades but rarely had time to put in the energy to be outstanding. Dwana, who lived a few houses down, became a fixture in his life beginning in high school. Dwana's parents were neglectful and emotionally abusive. She had indulged in the drug culture but was attracted to Tony's straight and solid presence. She ended up spending most of her free time at the Garcias'. It was almost as if she became one of the family members. Tony and Dwana began having sex when they entered high school. I thought, "This was his outlet." In her senior year, Dwana became pregnant. Tony felt extremely guilty about what he had done and didn't hesitate to ask Dwana to marry him. As a strong Catholic who regularly attended church with his family, it was the right thing to do.

"That is a lot of responsibility to take on. That must have been hard for you," I commented.

Again Tony replied, "Doc, I never thought twice about it. I felt bad getting Dwana pregnant. I really did care about her and so I married her. I didn't see any other choices." I sensed his guilt made the choice. It also fit the pattern of being a responsible caretaker who would sacrifice for others. Although

I understood the reason, my inner good guy felt queasy, as if he had fallen down through a trapdoor.

With Tony working full-time, Dwana became a full-time mother. They lived in the Garcia house, with the extended family helping care for their son Hector and the two children who followed in the first 4 years of the marriage. Tony continued working long hours as a mechanic while Dwana took care of the kids and helped the extended family with household chores.

Tony and Dwana saved money, and when they turned thirty they bought their first house, not far from his parents. Everything seemed good to those seeing them from the outside. Inside the marriage, there were the usual issues around money—not having enough of it—and the needy chaos of three young children. Without the extended family support, Dwana became depressed, withdrawn, and unresponsive to Tony. The couple stopped having sex. Dwana, who had had a petite figure in her early 20s, gained almost 80 pounds.

"How did you feel about Dwana being depressed and not willing to have a physical relationship with you?" I asked. To me, this suggested dysfunction in their relationship and a dangerous turn for Tony, who had few expressive outlets beyond his work. Dwana was obviously in some kind of psychological pain.

Tony shrugged. "Not much I can do about it. It is the bed I made for myself."

When Tony said this, the sick feeling in my stomach came back. I could feel his fatalism and resignation. I thought about how many people out there feel as if there isn't anything they can do with their lives. Perhaps I avoided my own depression by believing you can always take some kind of action. But something wasn't right in Tony's situation. I couldn't put my finger on it, but it made me want to offer a solution. This is usually not a great idea when exploring material. "You could do something, like go to couple's counseling or get Dwana into her own therapy to deal with her depression."

"I am here talking to you. That is something. I am hoping you can help me with my stress." He was right. He was taking action, and I was out of line, but his defensiveness around her depression and lack of sex troubled me.

"You are right. Tell me more about your life, Tony. Sorry to interrupt."

Tony seemed bothered by my comments. He seemed less engaged the rest of the session. I hoped we could start fresh when we met again.

In our next meeting, Tony described more about his job. Over the past several years, he began to work even longer hours, eventually becoming the owner of the auto repair shop. All of his energy went into building the business. He had upgraded the machinery, updated the computer software, and remodeled the bays and customer areas. Tony proudly pulled out before-and-after pictures on his phone. This was his baby, and he had poured his heart and soul into it. "That is impressive. You've really put everything into this." Tony smiled. I could tell it was one of his main sources of feeling worthwhile.

I brought Tony back to talking about his home situation. He told me that his kids were fine. His oldest was in the military, living abroad. His daughter was in nursing school, and the youngest daughter was in college. When they were young, he felt more relevant, but now "I am just their dad who loves them. They don't really need me except for the cash."

"What about your interactions with Dwana?" I asked.

"I try to ignore her negativity and stay positive, but the first things out of her mouth are complaints and bitches. I never hear, 'I'm glad you're home.'"

"I keep saying this, but Tony you are taking on a lot and not getting much back. I can understand how this might be stressful."

"Doc. If this is all it was, I don't think I'd be here." Tony had an edge, which is not uncommon in men who are depressed. Instead of overt sadness, it comes across as irritated or a little pissed off.

"You mean there is more?" I asked.

"Well, my dad has recently gone on dialysis for his diabetes. My mom is falling apart, so I have been taking off from work to help him out. I drive him for his treatments three times a week." He anticipated my reaction. "Before you say that's too much, I appreciate the time I get to spend with my dad. I know he is hurting, and it makes him feel better to have me there."

"That is admirable. It must feel good to be able to do something for your dad."

"Yes, it is. Unfortunately, it takes time, and it seems that I have no time."

"No time for yourself?"

"No time for anything. Everywhere I go, I feel like I am in a rush. I am afraid it will make me sloppy, forget important things. I deal with machinery, bills, employees."

As our second session ended, I sensed there was even more Tony needed to tell me. I felt a bit overwhelmed by the way he depicted his life. He was being so responsible with so little reward except for a successful business. I wondered how he was as functional as he was. It still wasn't adding up, but I worked with what Tony had given me.

## A Focus on Stress

Over the next several sessions, Tony talked in more depth about the stresses in his life, including being a business owner, son, parent, and his skeleton of a marriage. Just talking about it seemed to relieve some of his anxiety. We also discussed stress management techniques, including taking time to do mindfulness meditation at work twice a day and creating more efficient systems at his work to delegate responsibilities.

The most powerful conversation we had centered on self-care. Most dutiful men don't give to themselves the way they give to others. One of the lessons I had to learn in my life was self-compassion. This is the willingness to see yourself as your own best friend and treat yourself the way you would someone you really cared about. It wasn't until I went through a divorce that I was able to ask myself what I wanted to do rather than feed it through my partner.

"Being your own best friend? That seems pretty selfish," Tony countered.

"Selfish is bad?" I asked.

"Yes. You are putting your needs ahead of others. That runs counter to what I learned growing up at home and in the church."

"And how has that been working for you?" I asked in joking tone.

"What do you mean?" he replied, a bit defensive.

"I mean, you are the one who has been running around doing things for others and wearing yourself out. You don't sleep much. You worry. You are anxious. Seems like you could give yourself a little care. Would you consider that selfish?" I asked.

"What you say makes sense, but it feels very wrong. It is going to take some time for me to really buy into it. It is hard enough for me to walk away in the middle of the day to my office to do that silly 15 minutes of meditation you showed me. But I have to admit, I feel better. I feel like sometimes I can reset."

## Confronting the Shadow

Although I think I helped in a practical way with some of Tony's stress-related issues, his reluctance to address his primary relationship seemed a bit strange. I thought that with my support he would be more willing to push himself to work on the marriage. Without this discussion, it seemed as if we had reached a point where he didn't need my input. When I brought up the idea of tapering off our sessions during our eighth meeting, I fully expected him to let me know that he was done too. He looked at me and then dropped his head. I could tell that he was having trouble sharing his thoughts with me. Maybe he was more attached to our counseling than he had showed.

"So, I am feeling better. I have appreciated you listening and helping me with strategies to combat feeling so overwhelmed." Tony hesitated, and then added quietly, "There is one more thing I haven't talked about." He paused, and then continued, "When you started talking about our sessions maybe coming to an end, I thought I should probably bring this up. It is not easy." This was confirming my hunch that there was more to the story. I was curious. I anticipated it had to do with why he didn't want to work on his marriage.

"Of course. What is it?" I asked.

"This is difficult."

"Take your time."

"Well, there is this customer who I have known for a while. She and I have been pretty friendly over the years."

"What do you mean, 'friendly'?" I asked.

Tony hesitated before he answered. "It is hard to define. We have always had an easy time talking to each other. She has let me know about her life struggles. I have shared with her some of my stresses too. Well, about a year ago, I realized that I was more interested in her than just friends. I couldn't get her out of my mind. She is much younger than me, very attractive. She had made some suggestions that we should go out for dinner sometime. This was hard for me because as you know I am married, and have never cheated on my wife. I fantasized about being with her, but figured that was all it would ever be." This glimpse into Tony's fantasy life made him seem much more real. I sensed he was finally letting me in. Maybe the threat of me abandoning him in therapy was stirring it up. I took it as positive.

"Something has changed?" I asked.

"Yes. She and her husband split up about three months ago, around the time I started seeing you. She brought her car in and was a bit more forward than usual. I enjoyed the attention, and I know she did too. That night when she came to pick it up, she invited me out to dinner again. This time, she told me to meet her at her place. It was like a magnetic force field. So powerful."

"You couldn't resist?"

"Yes. It feels very weird talking about this. I never thought this would be my life. I went. We talked. We ate and then we made love. It was fantastic. But I felt horrible when I left. I was extremely self-conscious, as if everyone could see my transgression. I had never done anything like that before."

"You said this was around the same time you started coming to see me. Did this have anything to do with the overwhelming anxiety you were feeling?" I asked.

"Probably. But I was too ashamed to tell you or anyone about this." Tony paused for a few seconds. "I am in love with Brianna. I cannot get enough of her. I have been very careful about being seen, but yes, it is a big part of my stress. I feel embarrassed and ashamed. My parents would disown me. God has probably condemned me to hell."

Now the pieces made sense. Tony was already a guilt box, and now this. The overwhelming anxiety and the avoidance of relationship talk was all a part of trying to seal off this unacceptable aspect of him.

"How does it feel to have told me?" I asked.

"You've been pretty cool with me up to this point. It was getting harder to not tell you. I either had to just leave therapy or spill it. I guess I feel some relief."

The next session, Tony was a bit more forthcoming about his relationship with Brianna but reluctant to open up about his guilt and shame.

"This feels more like what I have been seeking in my life, someone who really wants to be with me. I just didn't think it was possible. We are really physical with each other. I told her about letting you know about our relationship."

"How did she react?" I asked.

"Brianna was relieved for me. She knew how much conflict I carried with me. It was an easier week. I think I need to start figuring out how to get out of my marriage."

"Before you go there, I wonder about the conflict part. I get that it is relieving to not carry around the secret, but it is still a secret to your wife, kids, and parents."

I wasn't sure if opening this up would be met by resistance. Tony had led a whole life in a good guy persona, and now he was face-to-face with the shadow part of himself. This part did not follow society's rules. It was pushing him toward getting his needs met. I was worried about how this conflict would play out in him. With his religious beliefs, shame, and guilt, I worried about self-destruction. What if the relationship with Brianna didn't work out? Then he would be left with himself, a flawed man, not the "golden boy" he had created for everyone else.

"Doc, I don't know if I can live with myself. I feel like just running off with Brianna and not turning around. Is that messed up or what?" he shared, not making eye contact.

"No. You've confronted a part of yourself that you have kept under wraps for a long time. I imagine that before Brianna, there were other secret transgressions which the 'good guy' might have kept secret." This was a hunch on my part, hoping that we could dive deeper than just this most recent incident of his hidden life. Tony's temple pulsed. His pupils dilated as he caught my gaze. Ten seconds passed.

"How do you know that?" he asked suspiciously.

"Tony, I don't know. I am just speculating given how much you have tried to do the right thing with Dwana, your family, and your business. All those times I have said, 'That's a lot' were because I thought you were being superhuman, too good."

Tony's chest started to heave. His cover was blown. I wanted him to break down here in the office, where I could support him, not alone with the moralistic internal judge to castigate him for his sins.

"I am so bad. I am so bad," he repeated as he started to sob, almost losing his breath. I let him release his shame without saying anything. I knew he had a whole childhood and adult life of trying to do the right thing. Any forbidden pleasures he indulged in were pushed quickly into some closed-off room in his consciousness while manifesting internally as guilt and self-condemnation.

Over the next several sessions, Tony revealed to me some of his most self-repugnant acts. We would spend each session focused on him examining the thought, the act, and the emotion. Rather than condemn him, I helped him understand the meaning. Slowly he began to apply the new paradigm to himself. In his mind, the Catholic Church and his parents didn't give him a way to be "bad" without being sinful. He started to see the connection to his self-image and secret life. In one of our sessions, he brought up a vice he has indulged in for more than 25 years.

"I'm not sure I told you about my late-night visits to the strip club," he shared.

"No. I'd like to hear," I said nonjudgmentally. My goal was to let him release his "sins," a bit like a Catholic priest but instead to an impartial Jewish psychologist.

"I still go sometimes, but it began when I turned 18, and I had found out that Dwana was pregnant. I sometimes would sneak off at 2 or 3 in the morning to a club not too far away. If she woke up, I would say I was just getting something to eat or that I couldn't sleep."

"Can you recall what you were thinking and feeling when you decided to make one of these runs?"

"You know, it was probably what we have been talking about. I felt like I had sacrificed so much for Dwana, my family, and my work that a part of me felt like I deserved to have some pleasure. By going in the middle of the night, it almost felt like a dream. Under the cover of darkness, I could sneak into the forbidden world. I went for a few hours and then came back before I had to get up."

"Seems like you got some satisfaction out of getting away with it," I said.

"You know. That's true. My shadow self, as we have been calling it, really dug going out into the night with a different identity. I was this other guy who could look at girls, have them interact with me, and enjoy my sexuality. I care about Dwana. She has had a really rough life, but I don't think I would have stayed with her if she hadn't gotten pregnant. There were other girls I was attracted to, but I felt obligated. I imagined that I could really be her savior . . . very 'Christ like.' That made me feel pretty righteous," he said, as he posted his arms up, as if he were on the cross.

"But obviously, you still had 18-year-old hormones and desire. There was bound to be conflict, but you didn't want there to be any," I commented.

"Right. So I locked away that night owl guy in my mind. He didn't exist to anyone else, except that he did for me. I just could never admit it."

"How is it for you to recognize him and maybe start to own him as a part of you?" I asked.

"Better than before we started talking about all this shadow stuff. It is hard for me now to imagine living this way. I guess all that stress I carried around was my own making. It's good to have a place I can try out accepting this part."

Six months into our weekly meetings, Tony broached the subject of leaving his broken marriage, but in a less frantic, reactive way. He was still dating Brianna. The frequency and intensity of their encounters had lessened, yet the relationship was developing in an authentic way.

"I think I'm ready to come clean with my family. I'm not so sure where this thing with Brianna is going, but I'd rather take that ride than the false one I have at home."

"What brought this up?" I asked.

"I've been thinking that I really don't want to live a double life anymore. When I am with Brianna, it feels good. I don't feel like I have to be exceptionally good, or be secretive. She was asking me about when I was getting out of the marriage. I am honest with her. I told her that I didn't know. But my lame answer stayed with me. I keep asking myself, if not now, when? I guess I need some help with this."

"What do you think keeps you from telling Dwana and your family?" I asked.

"I will really hurt them . . . bad."

"Let's break that down. Who is the 'them' you are most worried about hurting?"

"Even though I fear Dwana will flip out, we already live very separately. I think if she knew I would continue to support her financially, she might even be relieved. My kids are grown up. They see the dynamic at home and wouldn't be surprised. In fact, my son has asked me several times why I stay married to his mom when we don't really spend time together. He is pretty perceptive. My biggest fear is around my parents."

"Say more."

"They will feel betrayed by me. They thought I was this stand-up guy, but instead I am a lowlife who cheats and does bad things."

"That's your fear. What is the reality?" I queried.

"That is reality." I was surprised how quickly the internal judge took over Tony's psyche. I decided to confront that voice.

"Not from my angle, Tony. You have gone out of your way your whole life to be kind, supportive, and caring to your parents. You've described them as good Catholics. Is it realistic to think that they will throw all that you have done for them and your family away because you haven't been perfect?" Rather than name the sins, I was just trying to help him have some compassion around his imperfect self.

"What if they do? I'm not sure I could live without them. They are always there."

"They are not going to live forever, Tony. You would have to face the loss sometime. I am sure that your parents have not been perfect. This extreme anticipation of their rejection seems like it is more about your own shame than their condemnation." Tony didn't seem fully convinced. I continued, "So it sounds like it might not be so horrible to tell Dwana and the kids, but you are ashamed to let your parents know you aren't their perfect golden boy."

"Yes. I think telling them will be the hardest, but I need to do it. I am so tired of not being able to be honest with them or myself. Maybe you are right. Maybe they will understand that I am an imperfect sinner and that they can still love me."

"Can you say this to yourself? I am an imperfect sinner and I can still love myself," I stated as if I were him.

"You mean say this out loud here?"

"Yes. You know this is more about your own self-acceptance than anything else."

Tony squirmed in his seat. This was terribly uncomfortable for him. He was about to challenge the internal condemning judge in his own mind.

"Okay. I am imperfect . . ." He paused. "I know that." He laughed nervously.

"Say the second part," I implored.

"And I can still be okay with myself."

"Not quite ready to love yourself, but being okay with yourself is a step in the right direction. How does it feel to own this?"

"I am struggling to own it, Doc. I wish it was easier."

"You've had a lifetime of not believing it. It is going to take some practice." Our session was coming to an end. Tony shrugged as he rose from his chair to leave the office. "I can't wait for the day I really believe it. See you next week."

### Personal Reflection

- How do you feel about Tony's sense of duty and guilt? How might you approach this if you were his therapist?
- What are your reactions to infidelity? How do you integrate your own morals with the very human struggles that Tony describes?
- What are some of the potential cultural concerns that might make their way into therapy with Tony? How would you address them if you were his therapist?
- What are your reactions to the "shadow" as a way to understand some of Tony's secretive behavior?

### What Makes Tony a Good Candidate for Group?

In many ways, Tony had to take on adultlike responsibility at an early age. He pushed down the impact of not being able to be a "kid" and built a life around being dutiful. The internal conflict between trying to always be the good man and the secretive actions he took for his own benefit created a high level of stress in his life. Tony grew up with very traditional masculine and Catholic values. It was not acceptable for him to be a victim or to take time for himself. His duty as a man, father, husband, worker, and spiritual being took precedence over paying attention to his own needs and finding outlets to sustain himself.

In the men's group, he would be around some other guys who also understood the consequences of being the caretaker and responsible one. The give-and-take interaction in the group about topics that are not socially acceptable in other venues, like sex or infidelity, might help Tony begin to have more self-compassion, especially as he saw he wasn't the only one who wasn't perfect. The danger for Tony would be to become the group caretaker, replaying avoidance of his own issues to serve others. On the other hand, having honest male friendships might give Tony a more holistic perspective about what it means to be in relationships. By being encouraged to be real with his emotional life and confront his harsh inner judge, Tony might find a way to compassionately accept himself in the group setting.

# 6

# Questioning Identities

A stable adult identity is forged from life experiences that reinforce a consistent sense of self. It is not until one is confronted by unique life events that this identity is challenged. In this chapter, you will meet two men who have been shaken by life circumstances to question their identities. Peter is a survivor of a family tragedy that has made him question his religious upbringing and the nature of how he frames his life experience. Kean has had an intimate encounter with another man, leaving him confused about his own sexual identity. Through psychotherapy, each man navigates his past self and searches for new ways to define his current identity given the change of circumstances.

## PETER: LOSING MY FAITH

"I was always so sure of myself. I knew God was right there with me all of the time. He was my guardian. If I failed, there was always a silver lining that I should learn from. When I didn't get my way, I knew there must be a plan. But when Claudia and Lilly died, I just couldn't find a way to make it all right. I couldn't accept that God was trying to teach me some lesson. It woke me up," said Peter, who had consulted me as someone outside his faith community. Peter, a Caucasian man who wore wire-rim glasses, looked pale and sad. His body was pudgy and soft, as if he hadn't exercised in a while. Peter was in

http://dx.doi.org/10.1037/0000132-007
*Deepening Group Psychotherapy With Men: Stories and Insights for the Journey,*
by F. E. Rabinowitz

his early 30s and was 6 months into deep grief. His wife, Claudia, and his 2-year-old daughter, Lilly, had been killed in a car accident. Peter had sought help from his Fundamentalist church. Initially he attended counseling with his pastor and joined a grief group in the community, but his psychic pain had not decreased. In fact, he was feeling more agitated and angry. He dropped out of the grief group a couple of months into it and had not talked to his pastor in the past few months. Peter, who worked in his family's insurance business, was on partial leave. He had flexibility to come and go when he wanted and just maintained a few of his accounts. His parents, who ran the business, were supportive but were also a part of the religious community he was avoiding. Not wanting to face his former friends, neighbors, and coworkers, Peter had stopped socializing.

As a father and husband myself, I was not certain how I would have experienced the profound loss Peter had lived through. I immediately valued Peter's strength to reach out when most of us might just want to crawl in a hole and never come out. Although his pain was obvious, I thought it best to start with his own analysis of the "wake-up call": Had God abandoned him? Was it okay for Peter to abandon God—either temporarily or permanently? No longer was his religion a source of comfort or answers in light of the tragedy. I figured we'd get to the emotional part soon enough.

### Choosing Which Pain to Address First

To me, talking about faith and the lack thereof seemed like ground that might not be too overwhelming. I am Jewish by heritage and culture, and I rarely attend synagogue. And although I believe in the vast unknown, I find religion to be more of a narrative that originated as passed-down stories to help explain the mysteries of life. I was interested in how Peter would ask about and respond to my belief system.

"You lost your faith?" I asked.

"You could put it that way. It was more like I began to question everything I was taught in my life by my parents, the church, and the religious community."

"What specifically are you questioning?" I asked.

"Deep down, I am questioning whether God exists. When life was on a positive trajectory, I regularly attributed my extensive good luck to my belief in God. If I prayed and sacrificed for him, I would be rewarded with positive experiences. Everyone I knew seemed to believe this. We reinforced it with each other. If something challenging came up, it was God testing me. If I was scared, all I had to do was remember that God was watching over me, and I would relax and not worry."

"With the tragedy that happened, it is really hard to believe he was watching over you." I tried to empathize without judgment.

"This may sound sick, but you are one of the first people I have talked to who actually understands that concept. My pastor kept telling me that God had a plan in heaven for my wife and daughter. I should be happy that they are in this good place. I tried to buy it, but something told me that it was too easy an answer."

"It also did not give any validity to what you were feeling," I added.

Peter's eyes widened. His shoulders lifted as he moved up on his chair.

"Exactly. I was ripped apart. My whole world had been nuked, and this man of God was telling me I should be happy they were in heaven. What a crock!"

"It didn't fit," I responded, encouraging him to keep talking.

"No. It was so far from where I was, I just couldn't talk to him anymore. He's a nice enough man, but he was not there for me in the way I needed him to be."

"What were you needing?" I asked.

"That's why I am here, I guess. I saw your profile online and thought I need someone outside my circle to help me find the answers. You have a Jewish last name, and I have always respected the Jews for the way they question things. The Talmudic scholars were always pulling apart how to interpret events. Besides, the Jews have had to survive several Holocausts in the past 2,000 years, and somehow they are still around. Maybe your people know something about how to survive dark tragedy."

"I appreciate the positive association. You should know I am not much of a religious Jew. There are a lot of mysteries about life I don't understand, but I am someone who isn't satisfied with answers that don't make some kind of scientific, logical, or even emotional sense." I let him know where I was coming from. It felt honest, and if I am not a good fit, he should know that up front.

"Well, I could use some of that. Even the support group I went to was all about picturing loved ones in heaven. It felt like everyone was agreeing to believe in this idyllic heavenly place so that we could not feel our devastation. It was like 'let's pretend' that those we love are better off than they were with us."

"Sounds like that interpretation didn't resonate," I reiterated.

"I really wish it could have. Pretragedy, I would have bought it maybe. I would love to believe in this happy, peaceful, safe place in the sky that houses everyone who has died. But this horrible accident to two people who had a whole life to live . . ." Peter's eyes started getting glassy, and he sniffled. It was obvious he was trying to hold back tears.

"Peter, it is okay to cry here. That's why I have these tissue boxes around the room."

"I know. I'm used to crying privately. I was taught that real men don't cry. They stay strong. Crying is weak. So my whole life I have only cried alone. I'm pretty good at holding my tears back."

"Got it. Just know that if they do come, I do not see you as weak. To me, being able to cry shows strength. It is like you are free to feel whatever you are feeling."

"Appreciate the permission. Maybe I will get there. It is good enough to be able to talk without having someone tell me what I should be feeling."

At least Peter left the first session sharing and not being contradicted. At best, I reinforced the idea that he could talk about his pain, even if he couldn't fully express it physically. It might have overwhelmed him too much to cry in the first session in my presence. Many men who have been raised with traditional gender role norms inhibit themselves from showing vulnerable emotion, especially around other men they barely know. I had been prepared for him to unleash his frustration, anger, and maybe sadness, but it never really came. The existential questioning of God gave him a way to channel his confusing emotions. Even though he said he didn't believe in God anymore, he still used the idea of God be a guiding principle to his pursuit. When I went home, I hugged my wife and called my children, making sure they knew how much I loved them.

### Letting Him Choose the Path to Healing

In our next session, Peter looked as if he had been crying. His nose was red, his eyes watery, and his posture stooped. He sat down without making much eye contact.

"After our last session, I went home and cried for a while. I thought about Claudia and Lilly. I saw their faces. It was like we were sitting in our living room, just doing mundane stuff, like playing with dolls and talking about nonsense stuff that two-year-olds laugh at. It was surreal. I really broke down."

"You look like you were crying before you got here today."

"Very perceptive. Yes. Just thinking about coming here made me feel deeply sad. I sat in the car outside and just let some of my tears come."

"In here, you seem to have stopped," I said, still letting him know it would be all right for him to share his emotions in my presence.

"Yes. I still can't cry in front of anyone else. It feels very private. Sorry."

"No worry. What would you like to talk about today?"

"I'm not sure where to start."

"Anywhere is fine. Whatever comes to your mind first," I replied. Peter looked away for a few seconds, as if gathering his thoughts.

"I want to continue to talk to you about God." I was expecting him to want to continue to talk about the images of his wife and daughter, but perhaps the God conversation would be his way of getting there. Resolving his feelings about God seemed important to him. I just had to trust his unique process. This was going to be his path.

"Go ahead," I encouraged.

"When I was a boy, I looked up to all the adults. I was the oldest of my cousins but didn't have any siblings. I forgot to tell you that I was adopted. My parents couldn't have children, so they adopted me when I was a baby. I remember all of these outings we went on, usually involving our church community. We would go to church and then play and picnic. Those memories are beautiful. But now I am beginning to reconstruct what was actually going on."

"What do you mean?" I asked, interested in the adoption legacy. That alone is a very powerful dynamic—to know you biologically came from a different place than the one you were raised in.

"Well, I remember my parents and aunts and uncles saying that I was blessed and that God loved me. I took this in, and it did comfort me. I think they were probably talking about me being rescued from some poor teenage girl who gave me up for adoption. Of course, I ended up in a better place. I can only imagine the hardships I would have faced being raised by a 16-year-old. So in that sense I was blessed. But maybe I was just lucky. Maybe the 16-year-old and her parents thought it would be better for a baby to be raised by more mature people who really wanted him. When I think about it this way, God didn't really have to intervene to give me my parents."

"That sounds true. It might have just been a good decision for everyone involved," I restated.

"Exactly. No need for God to have this happen, yet I was constantly told that God had been the key to my life direction. It made me feel special."

"Special?"

"You know. It is like the Bible story of Moses being sent down the river and picked up by the Pharaoh's family."

"Yes. But you would also be special because you were a baby who was getting to live with loving parents."

"I know that, yet as I go through my life experiences I realize there were other ways I could have framed what happened to me."

I wondered where Peter was going with this. In a way, he was rewriting his personal narrative without the God part. This was something he could not do within the community. I felt as if I was being a witness to some kind of intellectual awakening. I just needed to listen and not judge.

"Dr. R., what do you think? I want your opinion about this. Could life be happening without any divine intervention at all? That would mean that we are here without any religious guideposts. While people who believe in their religion continue to think that it is God, maybe it's just random or at best unplanned consequences of actions."

### Connecting the Dots

"Peter, I am not a theologian. It looks to me as if you are doing what most good scholars and scientists do. They look at all of the possible explanations and find the ones that have the best data or logic behind them." We were going far afield from his feelings about the death of his wife and child. I was still hoping he would connect them. Maybe I was going to have to do that.

"So, Peter, how does this connect to your deep loss?" I asked.

Peter tilted his head and shut his eyes. He was silent. Something was going on in his head. I waited almost a minute before I asked what was going on with him.

"I'm considering the possibility that Claudia and Lilly's deaths were just bad luck. Claudia was driving on the freeway at the wrong place and time. When I believed God was in charge of everything, I thought that this could not happen if you were a believer. He would make sure that you were out of harm's way. But it makes me think that if God is not monitoring everything and everyone, then accidents can happen. You can be in the wrong place at the wrong time."

"Yes. That is possible," I agreed.

"Thank you for saying that." I'm not sure if I was being thanked because I validated his thought or because I didn't challenge it.

"Now I think I am ready to deal with my feelings. I just need to know that Claudia and Lilly were not the victims of God's wrath."

"Did you think God was punishing you by taking them away?" I asked, realizing that we had stumbled into Peter's guilt, a potentially huge emotional morass that could turn his pain inward toward self-contempt.

"Well, it crossed my mind. Maybe I did something that deserved that kind of punishment."

"Have you done something you feel horrible about?" I asked, realizing that he might be interpreting a correlation between his own actions and the deaths.

Peter hesitated and again shut his eyes. I waited.

"I have racked my brain a thousand times. I know I have been lazy off and on. I have not always appreciated the good life that I had. I could have done better in school. I have tried to be a good man, a good father, a good husband, a good son. Maybe I should have stayed home the day they were killed. I could have driven Claudia and Lilly to the doctor appointment they were going to. The timing would have been different, and maybe we would have avoided the accident." His eyes watered, but no tears.

"Yes. It might have changed the timing, but that doesn't make you responsible for their deaths. Sometimes holding on to a sense of responsibility is a way to feel some control in a situation that was out of your control. You couldn't follow Claudia or Lilly around every minute to protect them."

"I didn't think I needed to, because I thought God would care for them. I really did use God as a way to keep me from worrying about all the possible bizarre things that can happen. And then when it did happen, I wake up to a reality that I believed in a myth. How do people go around without a belief in God? This is really new territory for me."

"I hear that. It is a really different world without God watching over you and your loved ones. Yet you are still here, and you are surviving, as painful as it is."

"I think it is time for me to go," responded Peter, a teardrop hitting his pants leg. I nodded. It was the end of the session.

## Examining My Own Beliefs

Peter's story challenged me to look more deeply into my own beliefs. Was the universe ordered, or was it chaotic? Was there a divine being or beings overseeing this experience? If we are alone, what is the point of life beyond pure survival and propagation of the species? Why is the placebo effect so powerful? Belief in something can take away fear and doubt and allow us to do amazing and also brutal things in this life. Are we pack animals, like dogs or lions, interconnected by others, ensuring that we don't live or die alone? Do we continue to hold on to the childhood fantasy of omnipotent parents in the form of powerful authority figures and a concept of an all-powerful God? My head was spinning. I had read spiritual, psychological, and philosophical works throughout my life, and I had doubt about the strength of my beliefs. I was having trouble sleeping one night but had a vivid dream.

I was in a dark, foggy space, but there were astral beings floating around me. Like the roller coaster at Space Mountain in Disneyland that whips through the blackness, I was on a cosmic ride through a spirit world. There were images of my dad, who had died several years earlier, and of my grandparents, who had died even earlier. I saw what looked like the abstract figures of a Miró surrealistic painting. I felt as if I were being taken to the mythic river Styx. I was fascinated but also terribly sad. I began to weep in this ethereal world and couldn't stop. I felt myself dropping lower into the darkness. The ride was taking me where it wanted. I had no control . . . until I woke myself up. My face was wet with tears. I had cried, and it felt real, but what was it I had just experienced? Peter's painful reality slipped into my consciousness. Was I filling in the emotion he couldn't express? I hadn't felt deep sadness like that for a while. I anticipated Peter's session with a bit of trepidation. My dream not only dipped me into the world of grief and pain but also raised some questions in my mind about the nature of death. The dream was so vivid that it felt as if I had actually gone to some other astral plane. My rational mind quickly countered that my brain was fully capable of creating a simulation of an experience of spiritual transformation. But wasn't this the feeling that believers used to "know God"?

## Sitting With His Grief

Peter appeared for his session looking as if he hadn't slept much. His hair was uncombed. He wore a T-shirt and cargo shorts. His shirt had "Superman" written across it in the comic book font.

"So, Dr. R., I had this dream," Peter began. How ironic, I thought. Another coincidence? This work with Peter was starting to feel like not having a rudder in a rough sea.

"Tell me about it, Peter."

"Well, normally I don't remember my dreams, but this one was pretty vivid. Even you were in it." I nodded, curious about where this was going.

"I was walking along this river on a path by myself. The river was familiar but not someplace I can really point to. I look over into the water, and there is a boat with a group of refugees, like the ones fleeing the Middle East. At first I felt bad for them. They are heading upstream against the current. In the middle of the group, I spot my daughter, Lilly, sitting on a man's lap. She is staring out at the land without much expression. In the dream, I light up. I can feel it now."

"Say more about the feeling of lighting up."

"It is like someone opened the door to my prison cell after I have been condemned to life. A lightness of being. I am free to go. Pardoned."

"Wow. That is a powerful image."

"In the dream, I try to catch Lilly's eyes, but she is focused on something in the distance. I even wave to her, but the boat keeps heading up the river. I realize I am late for my appointment with you. Then I wake up."

"How did you feel when you awoke from the dream?" I asked.

"I felt relieved, like Lilly is still out there. It seemed very vivid. When I woke up I felt like it was a real experience, not a dream."

"How does it feel telling me right now?" I asked.

"Given our discussions about whether there is a God, it feels a little bit like a sign that maybe there is. It is making me doubt myself again. This time it feels like maybe I jumped too fast toward not believing. She seemed real in the dream, but then again it was just a dream. Right?" Peter looked at me, hoping I had a good answer. This was exactly the question I was hoping not to have to answer. My own dream had created doubt in me too.

"Dreams are still a part of the mystery of this life," I heard myself say, as if it were coming from someone else.

Peter nodded.

"What do you think, Peter?" I asked.

"I know the dream came from my mind, but it was stimulated by something real. It was comforting and a little disturbing. Maybe it is possible to embrace both. Life is pretty intense, but maybe there are layers to it. Today I feel deeply sad when I contemplate never being with Lilly and Claudia in the life we had. I mean, it is like a profound sad." Peter's voice trailed off. Tears came again. This time he started to weep in my presence. His chest heaved. I could hear the high-pitch sound coming from deep inside him. It was a wail that sounded like an aboriginal didgeridoo. I felt the tears in my eyes coming to the surface as well. I got goosebumps as I listened to his grief sing from his being. I sat with him for the rest of the session, handing him tissues.

"Thank you for sitting with me," he said as he noticed the time was almost up in the session. I nodded.

"Appreciate your realness and your trust with me. See you next time, Peter."

"Look forward to it, Dr. R."

## Personal Reflection

- What were you most moved by in Peter's family tragedy? How do you psychologically protect yourself from focusing on the potential losses of loved ones in your life?

- What are your beliefs about death? How have you handled deaths of friends and family in your life?
- What are the most important interventions a therapist can make when facing a man's grief? Was there anything you would have done differently in these sessions?

### What Makes Peter a Good Candidate for Group?

It was powerful to be in Peter's presence as he expressed a level of grief most of us hope never to experience around loved ones who died before their time. Peter is articulate, emotional, and at the same time stymied by his traditional male upbringing that emphasizes strong moral character and religious devotion. Although loss is a universal element of life, Peter has really been shaken to his core by losing the two most significant people in his life. Peter tried to be a part of a grief group, but the religious overtones did not capture what he was feeling. He was disillusioned to the point of almost giving up. The men's group, with its value on authenticity and connection, might have a much different response to his pain. Although most guys do what they can to distract themselves from loss, it is also the conflict zone that has direct access to the portal of depth. Peter needs support and understanding, but he doesn't need to be told how to do it.

The men's group would not be a good fit if it tried to problem solve his dilemma. It could potentially give him the safe space to feel his pain and allow him to hear other men's conflict, loss, and pain as well. The existential aspects of the men's group might help him see that there are alternative ways to interpret his life trajectory as well. Whereas some men might focus on Peter's intense story or religiosity to avoid being open to their own depth, his sharing may also have the effect of encouraging members to tap into deeper emotions around difficult elements in their own lives.

## KEAN: AWAKENED FROM CYNICISM

"I just felt like I was seen. I have never experienced that before. It was like the world became color from black and white. I want to get it back," pleaded Kean in our session. "I felt full, and like I deserved to be here and be loved."

Kean, whose mother was from Peru and father from Connecticut, had been in therapy with me off and on for 3 years and was describing a recent experience. I had never heard Kean talk like this before. He had a tendency to be morose about life. He was very smart but also super cynical. Kean was married to his college girlfriend. They had two children, both of whom were now in college themselves. The years of raising kids, which started just after both he and his wife graduated, Kean described as "total self-sacrifice." Kean had a comfortable managerial job at high-tech firm that had grown pretty stale. His initial consultation with me was to deal with his underlying depression, which he felt that he had inherited from his own father. Kean tended to use the sessions to complain about his life. His storytelling was engaging, but each had the theme of "life sucks." So when Kean came for his weekly session with a new attitude, I was suspicious.

### Something Has Changed

"Say more about this, Kean. I've never heard you utter those words before," I countered.

"I know it doesn't sound like me. This will certainly blow my chances for winning the cynic of the year contest again this year," he said with his usual self-deprecating humor.

"What happened to you?" I asked.

"I am glad that I have total trust in you, Fred, because I don't think I would ever talk about this. In fact, I am still pretty amazed about what I am experiencing. It feels more like a dream that is not happening to me. Well, you know I have been trying to get myself back in shape now that the kids are out of the house and I am pushing 45. I have been going over to the big fitness workout place on the west side of town every evening after work. Thanks to you, I have started to value my body more, and know that I have to take care of myself and beat my depression."

"So that has made you feel this good? That's great," I responded.

"No. That is great, but this is something else. As a part of my routine, I have been doing an exercise class with the music . . . you know, with the cheerleader workout guru yelling at us. You probably can imagine this room full of mainly middle-age women and me and this other guy. So Ben and I have been working out next to each other, cracking jokes about us being the only guys in the class. He has a similar way of humorously making fun of the world like I do."

"That's excellent that you have a made a male friend. We have been talking about how isolated you have been. How nice," I commented.

"Well. This is the part I thought would be easier to talk about, but it's not."

"What do you mean?" I asked.

"I guess I'll just say it. I really like this guy."

"Cool. What's so hard about saying that?" I asked naively.

"No, Fred, not he is a good guy, which he is, but I like him more than a friend. I can't believe I am saying this, but I'm feeling an urge to be with him."

"Urge?"

"You are making this hard for me. I am really into this guy and think he is really into me. Can you see the dilemma there, Dr. Psychologist?"

"You mean you are having romantic feelings?" I finally said, wrapping my head around this man, whom I had automatically put into the heterosexual box of sexuality.

"Yes. I said it. You heard me. I am glad we have confidentiality, because I have lived my whole life as a heterosexual man, and now I am feeling things that tell me that something else is going on."

"So you are feeling as good as you have ever felt, and it runs against your whole life narrative as a heterosexual man," I summarized for both of us.

"Bingo. Of course this is happening to me. All these years, I've been looking for the spark to break me out of my bubble of cynicism, and this is the answer?" Kean shook his head but still had a smile on his face. "No, it couldn't be some lifestyle changes that gave me a new perspective on life, it had to be a 'gay' thing. As you know, I have no problem with anyone being gay, but I did not see this coming."

"So you are conflicted because it feels so good, but it runs counter to who you thought you were?" I asked.

"Yes, but no. I am totally who I am with Ben, and he gets it. He sees me. He appreciates me in a way that I have never been appreciated before. Hannah, God bless her, has put up with me for over 20 years as her depressed, deadpan humorous husband. I have been pretty asexual, even though she has tried. Maybe this has been there the whole time."

"Maybe. Had you ever had fantasies about other men or experiences with guys?" I inquired.

"I was always the little guy growing up, youngest of five kids. You know my story of my parents' divorce when I was 6. When Dad left, my mom went into a tailspin. Dad rarely came by. He gave her custody of all of us, and we lived pretty poor. I was the young, naive one who would constantly hope that Mom would snap out of her depression. In fact, I was her baby and tried to cheer her up. We've talked about my cynicism being born out of failed hope. I was always hoping it would be better, but as each of my siblings left, I felt even more burdened."

"Yes. That is a breeding ground for a loss of hope, especially when it doesn't get better," I added.

"Then Dad commits suicide when I am about to go to college. I heard about it from my older sister, and we never talked about it. Even though I didn't have good feelings about him, it was the nail in the coffin, literally, for ever feeling good again. You know that story. Did I answer your question?"

Kean normally would have gone into a very dark place in mentioning his father's suicide. Today it seemed as if he was not dipping into those waters. I noted that and responded, "Not really, but I do appreciate what you are saying about understanding your cynical nature, but I asked you about feelings toward other males in your life."

"Oh yeah. I dodged that question pretty well. What would you call that . . . unconscious forgetting? Anyway, I did have some experimentation when I was little. During the chaos of Mom and Dad splitting up, my older brothers became my guardians. The three of them included me in their play, and there were some times when some of their friends did some touching and had me do the same. I didn't think much about it because I was pretty much 'hetero' in my orientation. I thought about girls, and when I met Hannah in college, I was pretty sexually active with her. I don't know if the fooling around as a boy opened the door? These days they talk about being fluid in sexuality. Maybe that's me. I don't know."

## Seeking Connection and Validation

"How do you make sense of the way you are feeling with Ben?" I asked.

"I don't know. I just know I'm out of my depression. He understands me, but also there is something about him that makes me feel good about being me. It feels sexual, but if he was just a good-looking guy, I would notice but not feel compelled to do anything about it. It's the connection that combines with the attraction. I've never felt this before. Anyway, you can imagine that I haven't said a word to Hannah about this. I'm not sure what to say."

"You still don't seem so sure what it means for yourself yet. How do you imagine Hannah reacting?" I inquired.

"We have been pretty separate lately. She's been pretty busy at the hospital, doing extra nursing shifts. The more I talk about this with you, the more I realize I am going to have to first make sense of this for me."

Kean and I continued our regular meetings, trying to unravel the changes in his life. Even though Kean had been coming for therapy for almost 3 years, the relationship with Ben had stirred up the most in-depth self-analysis to this point. He had been reviewing his childhood, his dynamics with each of his siblings, and his parents. Kean's mood remained positive, even as he explored questions about his sexuality, his isolation, and his long-term relationship with Hannah. In the eighth session after talking about his friend Ben, I helped him question what this relationship may really be about.

"I'm not sure that Hannah really sees me anymore. I think I am just her 'take it for granted husband.' My body has gotten into really good shape, and she hasn't even noticed. In fact, I have been overtly more sexual with her, more energetic in our interactions, and it has gone nowhere. Even though there hasn't been anything physical with Ben, he comments about how good I am looking physically and seems to be more attuned to who I am as a person."

"Sounds like you are playing off the energy you are getting in your interactions with Ben and trying to channel them toward Hannah."

"Yes. But she is not used to me being like this. Either she is totally clueless, or she doesn't know what to do with me. I have been more positive, and not depressing at all. You would think she would notice."

"You sound a bit pissed off that she is not," I replied.

"I am pissed off. I thought if I was not depressed, she would like that. Instead I feel like I am in an alternate universe with Ben. He totally notices me, we make direct eye contact, and we can talk about everything from politics to history. I do wonder what's in it for him."

"Have you talked about that?" I asked.

"No, not really. I don't even know if he is actually gay. It seems that way, but neither of us has made any moves. I know he is single and not currently in a relationship, but I don't want to make him uncomfortable by talking about it. We see each other every day at exercise class and occasionally get together for lunch, but other than that I just know he works for some insurance company. I'm pretty curious about his background, given I don't know that much."

"You asked what's in it for him, but I wonder what's in it for you? You are in a long-term relationship, yet the way you talk about this is more like an affair you are having," I interpreted.

"I know. I think I am just getting the validation I have never felt like I got from family or even Hannah. I'm not sure what else is going on, except me questioning my sexuality, which is a big deal, but for some reason I am not afraid."

"Interesting for you to feel so good and not be focused on what might happen to your marriage and your family," I commented.

Kean shrugged as the hour ended. "I'll think about it."

### Learning to Become His Own Friend

The following week, Kean looked different. I had gotten used to seeing him happy and excited about his life and the relationship with Ben. He plopped in the chair and let out a sigh. Kean shook his head from side to side, looking a bit like the old depressed Kean.

"I knew it was too good to be true," he said with exasperation.

"What happened, Kean?" I asked.

"Ben. He wasn't at exercise class this past week. Not a big deal, but I did try to text him and got the message kicked back to me. He no longer has the phone number."

"No explanation?"

"No. I did not see this coming. Last time we saw each other was last week after our session. He and I did our usual class and then went and had a drink after at a local pub. Again, no warning that he was leaving or heading out of town. Maybe I'm overreacting."

"It's really going against the pattern you had set over the past few months. Sounds like you are taking this personally."

"Well, yes. We had gotten pretty close as friends."

"What makes you so sure it is about you? Maybe there is another explanation that you just don't know," I added.

"Maybe, but something is really strange. I checked out the business where he worked. I called over there, and they were very cautious about even acknowledging he ever worked there. It was like they thought I was a nutcase, or maybe he never did work there. Things aren't adding up."

"You are having a strong reaction. What is his disappearance stirring up in you?"

"It's a feeling like the rug got pulled out from under me or when Charlie Brown is about to kick the football and Lucy picks it up. I let my guard down, and this is so sudden."

"Like you should have seen it coming?"

"Maybe. It's more like I didn't use my usual distancing techniques and now I'm exposed and hurting. I hate that."

"You feel sucker punched."

"Yes. Fuck him. But something was there. Now I feel foolish like a naive schoolboy. He played me like when I was a kid with my brothers."

"Did something happen between the two of you the last night you saw him?" I asked, wondering if there was some clue that Kean may have overlooked.

"Not that obviously comes to mind, but I have been obsessing about it."

"What did you talk about?" I asked.

"Stuff about the class. We talked about maybe doing something in the future. . . . Wait, that was a new conversation. I mentioned maybe going to the beach, and Ben got a little quiet. Maybe I came on strong. I still don't know if he is gay. Shit, I don't know if I am gay. This is all confusing me."

"Let's take it one step at a time. Where do you want to start?" I asked.

"I want to know why being with this guy got me out of my depression."

"What do you think, Kean?"

"I wonder if maybe I am gay and this whole life of mine has been on lockdown because I was afraid to admit it. I couldn't ever take the risk. With Ben, I felt comfortable, even though we never got physical."

"How does that feel as an explanation?" I queried.

"I'm not sure I believe it. My fantasy life has always been fairly heterosexual. Something about the connection and acceptance penetrated me more than I could imagine."

"I wonder if there is something that Ben represents in you? Like a part of your own psyche that you haven't been able to access?" I asked.

"I have always been really critical of myself, and when I was around Ben, that voice seemed to go away. Are you saying that it's not really Ben but actually me that is allowing myself to be comfortable to be who I am?"

"Does that make sense to you?" I asked as our time ran out.

"Yes. I probably need to think about it more, but I want to believe that I do have that power," he said as he rose from his chair to leave, less agitated than when he entered the session.

Kean cancelled his session the day before our next meeting with a short message that he was too busy at work and would keep his next appointment. I was surprised but also aware that he might be hesitant to challenge himself in our session. I was worried that he was still attributing too much to Ben and not enough to himself. Ideally, therapy should be a way for him to own his own power to decide how he views himself and others. I also thought about the sexuality question. I was open to the possibility that he may be gay, be bisexual, or have a fluid sexuality, but I also know that for many men, intimacy has been associated with sexuality. It is easy to confuse feeling comfortable around someone with being attracted to him. Kean seemed genuinely less depressed and more open when the relationship with Ben was conflict free. Now that there were some issues, I wondered if he would regress to his prior cynical style.

Kean did appear for his next session in his gym clothes. We made small talk for a little while before Kean dove into what had been driving him.

"I just worked out before I came over tonight. I thought it would be good for me to go there, and then talk with you. I have been regularly working out, even though I have not seen Ben at all since we last talked."

"What has that been like?" I was curious as to how he was processing the abandonment of this friendship.

"I have tried to take what we talked about a couple weeks ago about giving myself what I thought Ben was giving me in terms of self-acceptance and acknowledgment. It hasn't been easy. With Ben, it was almost like doing a drug that had immediate impact. I still can hear the critical voices wanting to squash that positive image I am trying to hold on to."

"I hear your struggle, but it sounds like a great start to not giving away your power. Reversing years of seeing yourself one way takes time to take hold, but at least you recognize the voices," I added.

"Yes. Once I realized that the whole Ben infatuation thing was probably something I created in my mind, I did reflect on what we talked about. If I can make him take away my cynical self, then I should be able to do it for myself. This is what I want to work on in our therapy."

"That's a huge step. How have you been making sense of the sexuality piece?" I asked, sensing Kean's openness with me.

"That part is still not so clear. At the gym, I have been noticing who I am attracted to, and it seems like I see attractive people everywhere, male and female. It makes me think that perhaps I'm not so pigeonholed in that realm. I still feel attraction to Hannah but have been hesitant to tell her about my inner life, given how weird it has been."

"What makes you hesitate?"

"I don't know. I guess I am afraid that she won't support my 'new' self-image."

"What makes you believe that?" I asked, trying to challenge his static vision of his long-term partner.

"I think she is just used to me being cynical and not very open. I think she has adapted to it, and so it would probably throw her off. She'd think I had lost it."

"What would be worst-case scenario if you did reveal a more positive you to her?" I asked.

"When you say it like that, I think maybe she would be more positive in response to me, but so far she hasn't really noticed. Maybe I'm afraid it wouldn't matter to her."

"That sounds like what drives your cynic," I noted.

"You mean my fear that nothing will change makes me cynical, like a defense against being disappointed?" Kean had a look that told me he was actually integrating the cognitive and emotional elements of his character. After a few seconds of looking blank, he broke a smile. "We have probably talked about this before, but it feels different this time. I actually believe it in my body. Being in touch with my fear is a little scary, but I at least feel something. In my cynic state, I am hard and not really touched by life. It is a good protection."

"Yes. It is good to protect you but not so productive in terms of growth and being more open," I reflect back to him.

As Kean stood up to leave, his face was more animated. He turned before he left and said, "This is going to need more practice, but at least the door is open. It was easy with Ben, but then it was probably safe because he didn't know me outside of the gym. Next step is to be more open with Hannah. I will let you know how it goes."

I nodded. I felt more confident that he had turned a corner, and I figured he would have a hard time turning back on the journey, even though it would be a treacherous one.

### Personal Reflection

- What was your initial reaction to Kean's shift from cynical to engaged? What was it about the relationship he had with Ben that seemed so life changing?
- What was your reaction to Kean's confusion around his sexuality? How would you have handled the discussion about sexual orientation?
- How did Kean's childhood experiences make him vulnerable to depression?
- How have you dealt with low periods in your life? Where do you get your support and validation when you are feeling down? How might this inform how you work with depressed individuals?

### What Makes Kean a Good Candidate for Group?

Early childhood chaos, possible abuse, and loss have left Kean vulnerable to depression and self-hatred. He has had to take care of himself and learned to not expect much, as he has been disappointed multiple times in his life. This wounding provides him with a portal to his emotional depth and fears about what it might be like to stop using his defense system to distance himself from others. Although his cynical stance keeps him at arm's distance from most of his relationships, the connection with Ben seemed to break through his usual defenses and create a conflicting wrinkle in his long-standing relationship paradigm. The encounter at the gym seemed to spark a willingness to be more open and engaged with others.

The men's group might provide a safe space for Kean to develop relationships with other men. To be able to talk frankly and get honest feedback about his cynical distancing methods might allow Kean to internalize a sense of self-acceptance. It is possible Kean might hold back from the group, given his trust issues. More likely the group might benefit from Kean's articulation about distrust while being supportive of his efforts to take risks to be real within the group. Kean seems ready to be seen as he is and to be supported in his efforts toward self-improvement and honesty with himself.

# 7

# The Perils of Addiction

Freud (1910) believed that seeking pleasure is a strong motive for human behavior. Although most of us find safe outlets to escape psychological pain, there are some whose lives are derailed by addiction. Addiction can be seen as repetitive, compulsive behavior that negatively impacts productivity, learning, and interpersonal relationships. In this chapter, you will meet two men who manifest their addiction in different ways. Carlton, a survivor of trauma, has found drugs, alcohol, and food to be pleasurable substitutes to feeling his emotional pain, even to the point of being life threatening. Neil finds the intoxication of new romantic relationships such a driving force in his life that he has difficulty maintaining intimate, genuine connections with others. Through psychotherapy each man struggles to confront the internal factors that contribute to his addictive drive.

## CARLTON: SLOW-MOTION SUICIDE

Several men I have known have committed suicide. It is the ultimate act of someone who wants out of the life he is living. Sometimes it is a dramatic event designed to punish others. Other times it is private. The latter is often accompanied by a hope that he will not be missed, that he can just fade away, denying his impact on those who love and care for him. There are 117 suicides every day in the United States. More of them are men than women. White men

http://dx.doi.org/10.1037/0000132-008
*Deepening Group Psychotherapy With Men: Stories and Insights for the Journey,*
by F. E. Rabinowitz

account for seven of 10 suicides (Centers for Disease Control and Prevention, 2015; Phillips, Robin, Nugent, & Idler, 2010). In my clinical work, I often come across men who are engaged in what I call "slow-motion suicide," which is much more common than the active variety. Slow-motion suicide is long-term self-destructive behavior that accumulates and often accounts for a shorter life span for men than women. The self-destruction occurs one day at a time in the form of testing death. It might be the amount and quality of food he eats. It is contained in habits like smoking, unsafe sex, driving fast, drinking too much alcohol or doing drugs, and not getting health checkups. Many men kill themselves slowly, usually only noticeable to those who care about them. It is a way to say, "I don't care. I will do what I want and deal with the consequences later." The later consequences are premature death through accidents, preventable diseases, and loneliness.

Carlton, 44, had never before been to therapy but came as a favor to his buddy, who he said was worried about him. Carlton was a massive individual in all ways. He was at least 6 foot 5 inches and more than 350 pounds. He lumbered into the office, ducking through the door, and then hesitated about where to sit. He had to decide between a chair that might not support him and a couch that might be hard to get up from. Carlton decided on the leather couch, took what seemed like a large gasp of air, and hit the cushions with a thud. He was a light-skinned African American with gentle eyes and a pleasant, nonthreatening smile.

"So how does this work, Doctor?" Carlton started. I could sense his discomfort with everything about this setup, from my Jewish sounding last name to being coaxed into talking to a white guy about his problems. I tried to ease the transition.

"First of all, I appreciate you making it in to check this out. It is not easy to come see a psychologist. Feel free to call me Fred. Carlton, this is an opportunity for you to look at yourself and work on any changes you'd like to make, with the help of an experienced guide. As you read in the paperwork, everything that goes on here is confidential and will never be shared outside of this room. Only situations where you are in imminent harm to yourself or others or instances of child or elder abuse are subject to breaking confidentiality for your own or others' protection."

"I still am not sure what to do. My friend Matt told me about you and thought it would be worth my time to talk."

"I would be interested in hearing your story." Rather than ask a list of questions, I like to find out about a man from the way he talks about his life. I can pick up on the nuances in his expression, as well as the content.

"My story? Like my whole life? Where do I start?"

"Start anywhere you want. I'm interested in why you think your friend thought it might be a good idea to talk with me."

"You know Matt. He is a worrier. He and I have been friends since high school. We met playing on the football team. He was the kicker and I was, as you might imagine, on the offensive line. Anyway, life doesn't always go the way you want it to."

"What do you mean?" I asked.

"You know, you have fantasies about the future and what it might bring and then there is the reality of life."

"What were some of your fantasies?"

"Nothing too extravagant. I wanted to have a family . . . wife, kids. I wanted to have a good job, a house, and be happy."

"Sounds reasonable. What happened?" I asked, curious about the reality of life he had mentioned.

"How much time do we have?" Carlton cracked the big grin. I figured that joking was one of the ways he deflected painful emotion.

"We have the rest of this hour and whatever else we decide in the future."

"Man, you do this for a living? I can't imagine how much crap you must hear. Must be depressing." I could sense another deflection. I expected this given that he had been prodded to come rather than looked forward to it.

"I actually appreciate the struggle that we all go through and know that for a lot of guys, the real story never gets told," I shared.

## Getting Real

Carlton hesitated before responding, as if he was trying to assess how to handle this situation sitting across from me. I imagined that he was having to make a decision about how real to be. Most guys want to present themselves in the best way possible and not expose their shame to the light. I sensed that Carlton was calculating how to best do this.

"I haven't really accomplished any of my goals. I talk a good game, but I have not achieved anything."

"Anything?" I asked.

Carlton leaned in and looked me in the eyes. No smile. Just anguish. "Look, man, I am single, never married. What chance do I have of having a family at my age? Look at my size. What woman would want to be with me? I live with my mother in our small little house in a crappy neighborhood. My job is basically a card dealer and professional gambler . . . not exactly big bucks and stable. I also have a damn cigarette habit. I drink too much and probably smoke too much dope. That pretty much sums up why I will never get anywhere near my fantasy of a normal life." Carlton had an edge, and he pulled it out to push me away. Presenting himself as a lost cause might end this little rendezvous he did for his friend.

"You sound like you have given up," I responded, not biting too hard on the hopelessness, putting the responsibility back on him.

"You could say that. I get what I can from this life. I'm not sure how much longer I am going to be here. Look at me. I am now officially diabetic, and you know that doesn't end well. My heart is probably messed up. I did get myself off of meth several years ago, but all that did was make me even more of a glutton to stuff my face full of food. I am probably not worth your time."

"You say probably. A part of you showed up today because maybe there is some hope in there somewhere," I countered, fully aware that Carlton was unlikely to act on it. My only chance was really to turn up the heat. This might be the opening to jump-start some lifestyle changes.

Carlton looked away and sat back on the sofa. I imagined that I had somehow penetrated his usual defenses. He tried to push me away with a "look how messed up I am" narrative. His identity as a failure exposed, I was offering him a way out. It was maybe a long shot, but he had told me he was a gambler. He let out a sigh. "You are right. I did show up today. I did it for my friend, but maybe it was the excuse I needed to get some help."

"That's okay. You are here." We spent the rest of the first session going over his history, including some discussion about his early family life. Carlton was the youngest of seven children. His dad was African American, his mom Caucasian. His father was a steelworker who lost his job when the plant closed down. He died from a heart attack when Carlton was 10 years old. His mom raised the kids and went back to work as a secretary when his dad became unemployed. During most of his childhood, Carlton's older sisters cared for him. Given his mother's schedule, they were responsible for cooking and cleaning when they got home from school. Carlton did not have much structure at home but did excel at sports. His size made him a valued player on the basketball and football teams. Carlton looked back with great fondness on his high school years, when he was popular and successful.

"That was the last time I felt confident in myself and that I might actually have the kind of life I wanted."

"What happened?" I asked.

"I was ready to go to the local community college. That was all we could afford. My older brother got himself in trouble. He was busted for robbery and ended up in prison. One of my sisters got hooked on drugs. My mother lost her job, and I got caught in all of the drama. I couldn't concentrate on schoolwork, so I dropped out and took a job at the local casino as a chip runner. I helped out at home but lost my way. I started smoking dope and doing some gambling. Pretty soon my life was sucked down the drain at the casino and the guys that hung out there. We played cards, craps, and engaged in some illicit activity that I am not proud of."

"Seemed like a lot was going on with your family and maybe this was an escape from that?" I ventured.

"I just lost my focus. College got further and further away. I went from being a stud physically to being a big, fat man. The other guys started calling me 'Pudge,' and I accepted it as an identity. I think I used it to let me be a glutton . . . for everything from food, to alcohol, to gambling, to sex, you name it. I am still Pudge to everyone in that group of friends."

"How about your friend Matt?" I asked.

"Matt and I still occasionally hang out. I think he is the only one from high school I see. Matt has stuck by me, even though we have gone in very different directions. Matt is a high school principal at an inner-city school.

We meet every few months for dinner. He is a genuine person. I look up to him. He has tried to help me out and has probably saved my life a few times. He bailed me out of jail once, and he also paid for me to take a vacation to Hawaii so I could get out of a jam with some underworld guys."

"He really cares for you. What was happening when he recommended you come and see me?" I asked.

"We just sat down to get something to eat and I lost it with him. I told him how much of a failure I was and that I didn't see much point in continuing. I was ready to just take a bottle of pills or put a gun to my head. He listened, was supportive but also gave me your name. Told me he'd pay for it. I guess I did need it."

"You open to coming back next week for another meeting?" I asked, as our time wound down.

"A part of me still thinks I am a lost cause, but I'm also a gambler. If there is a chance, I should probably give it a try."

### Gambling on Making a Change

I thought about Carlton and all that he had been through. He did have a lot of the qualities of some of the guys I knew who had committed suicide, but he also had some positives that might give him a chance to have a decent life. He was intelligent and had access to his internal thoughts and emotions. Carlton's friend Matt was in his corner, and I think the reason Carlton was still here is because of that support. On the other hand, Carlton had dug a pretty deep hole. Change was not likely to happen quickly, and because of his pattern of opting for immediate gratification, this would not be easy. I figured if he could gamble, so could I, despite the odds.

Carlton made it to our next meeting. He still had the big, friendly smile upon entry, but he soon got serious once we continued his life story. I could sense that the telling of the tale was therapeutic in itself and that he was willing to roll the dice on the process of getting some help. Because his friend was paying for the sessions, he also had some sense that Matt's support was real and that Carlton had some obligation to try to make it work. Any motivation is positive when trying to make life changes.

"I was thinking about what we talked about last time. I think the thing I am the most ashamed of was that I haven't been able to figure out how to do life right," Carlton shared.

"What do you mean 'right'?" I asked.

"I look at Matt. I look at you. You guys figured out the rules and took advantage of the system and now you have what you want. I have not done that. I can make excuses. That's what I do."

"What kinds of excuses do you make?"

"I say that I had a crap childhood. I can say that being African American puts me at a significant disadvantage. I can say that I probably am too impulsive, so I get distracted from my long-term goals with immediate gratification.

Finally, I am just lazy. No one can do it for me. I have to step up. Even when I get some kind of edge, I get in my own way every single time."

"You have some examples?" I asked.

Carlton thought for a few seconds. He looked down at the ground as he began to speak. "Yes. I had a chance last year to move up into a management position at the casino. Right now I am a dealer in the poker room. It pays okay, but I do the same thing every day without much to look forward to. My boss approached me. He has seen me do this job for years. I think he was trying to help me out. So I thought about it, and got excited. Then I got a bit freaked out. I would have to supervise people, watch the money, and report to the high-level managers. I would also have to dress up and be 'the adult' in a room full of impulsive gamblers. The night before the interview, I guess I self-destructed. I ended up going out with my crazy friends, drank too much, smoked too much, and got home around 6 a.m. pretty messed up. My interview was at 9. I passed out and woke up around 4 in the afternoon. I had text messages from my boss trying to find out what happened. Once I realized how late it was, I just called in sick since I was supposed to do my regular shift at 5 p.m. I didn't even mention it when I got back to work. I just acted it like it didn't happen. Great way to move up the ladder, huh?"

### Confronting Fear and Shame

"What were you afraid of, Carlton?" I asked him directly.

Carlton hesitated before responding, as if he was trying to access some kind of insight but it wasn't there for him.

"I don't know. I just think I'm a pathetic loser. What do you think, Doc?"

"From your story, it sounds like you were afraid of what success might mean for you." I paused and let that sink in, then added, "What are your thoughts about that?"

"Yes. I think it was a great opportunity for me to fail. There, I said it."

"So you would rather just not try to avoid being in a failure situation?"

"Exactly."

"Shame is pretty powerful motivator," I shared.

"Damn right. Every time I imagine making a move, I end up thinking, who do I think I am. Everyone is going to see me for who I am. Even if I succeed a little, it is only a matter of time before I am found out for the loser I am. Better to lay low and avoid."

"At least you know what your tendencies are," I said in a supportive way.

"Yes. I wish I didn't. It is hard for me to have any hope when I know it is all going to end bad anyway. Might as well indulge myself with some pleasure since I can't seem to sustain anything else."

"It is like you have a shame cloud that follows you around. It's hard to find any clear sky." I reframed the shame as a metaphor to give him something tangible with which to work.

"Good way to put it. How do I destroy the shame? Is it even possible?" Carlton asked with genuine interest.

"I'm not sure about destroying the shame. I think it is more about understanding it . . . figuring out what is its function," I responded.

"What do you mean *function*? It seems like it just keeps me down."

"Well, I wonder if the shame protects you from what it perceives as potential hurt. By keeping you out of challenging situations, you are safe," I interpreted.

"Safe and lame. Nothing good ever happens. I just sink deeper. Now I am 44. I wish I could go back in time and finish college. Eat right. Find someone who could love me."

"Why do you have to go back in time for that? You could start today," I say with a bit of "rah-rah" encouragement.

"Right. Look at me. Look at my life. Who would want any piece of this?" Carlton stated with conviction, putting a hand on his large stomach.

"You seem pretty sure, Carlton."

"I may be a gambler, but I am also realistic."

We were running over time, so I let Carlton know we would pick up from this point next time. He thanked me for listening. I was worried about the heaviness of his self-loathing, but at least he was saying it out loud, making it open for some kind of challenge and modification through our therapy.

### Responding to the Crisis

Before our next session, I got a phone call from Matt, who said that Carlton was in the hospital and wouldn't make the next session. He had been involved in a fairly serious car accident. The details were a bit fuzzy, but it seemed that he had been driving home around 2 a.m. from the casino and had been hit going through an intersection. He was not wearing a seat belt. Matt asked if I would be willing to do a session in the hospital with Carlton when he was in better shape. Without prompting, Matt said he had noticed that Carlton had been more truthful with him as a result of the counseling sessions with me. Because of confidentiality, I didn't say much, but I thanked Matt for letting me know what had happened.

Three weeks later, I was finally able to see Carlton in the hospital. I got the nurses to give us some confidential space in his room. Carlton was tilted up in his hospital bed. He had a cast on one of his arms. He had an intravenous tube in his other arm. One eye was partially swollen shut. He recognized me when I walked in the room. I could see an attempt at a smile, but it looked painful.

"Hi, Doc. Almost did myself in, but I'm still here," Carlton tried to joke.

"Looks pretty messed up," I said.

"No kidding. Lying in this bed has given me time to think about life and death."

"Anything you want to share?"

"I know you won't judge me, but it is still hard to be real, even with you."

"Do your best," I encouraged.

"I think I might have been wanting to die the night I got in the accident. It had been a shitty night at work. There were some rude, racist players who were making fun of everyone, including me. Usually I just blow it off, but it got to me. These privileged assholes were stiffing me on tips, calling me 'boy,' and complaining about what a bad dealer I was. I held it in and didn't show them anything."

"You must have been feeling a lot of anger."

"I was angry, but then also angry at myself for having put myself into this kind of situation in the first place. If I had gone to college and lived up to my potential, I wouldn't be in a position to take their crap."

"So you were beating yourself up. Turned the anger inward."

"So when my shift was over, I went and had a couple of drinks at the bar in the casino before jumping in my car. I felt a little looser. I don't remember much about the accident. I remember cranking music in my car and driving pretty fast. The next thing I knew, there was a cop trying to talk to me, and an ambulance ride. Then I just woke up here. I had no idea where I was, or even what day it was."

"Wow. You are lucky to be alive," I said.

"Lucky or unlucky? I want to see it as some kind of Lady Luck giving me one more chance, but maybe I am just continuing my bad run in this life." I ignored his self-deprecating comment and focused on the optimism I heard in what he was telling me.

"What do you want to do with the chance you have been given?" I asked.

"You are reading my mind," replied Carlton. "I've been thinking more seriously about making some changes. Ha. I've probably dropped twenty pounds in the past month from not being able to eat. It's a start." He smiled.

"What other changes have you been thinking about?" I asked.

"I want to go back to school. I want to get my bachelor's degree. There is some structure in doing that. Matt was telling me that a lot of schools now have online courses and weekend courses designed for people like me, who are returning."

"That sounds really positive."

"And I want to quit drinking and smoking. That stuff just keeps me from achieving anything."

"That's a lot. Do you have a plan for how to quit?" I asked.

"You asked me what I was thinking about changing. I'm going to need some help. I'm hoping we can continue to meet. Maybe we can figure out some ways to move beyond my tendency to self-destruct."

"I'm open to exploring all of that with you," I responded. Carlton started to nod out, his open eye shutting. I knew that the accident that almost killed him was responsible for his current desire to change. But sometimes, it is coming face-to-face with the reality of death that makes one reconsider the game plan. I was willing to be a guide on his long journey back.

"See you soon, Doc," he whispered as I walked out of the hospital room. I turned around and smiled. "See you soon, Carlton. Make sure you call when you are out." He gave me a thumbs-up with his nonbroken hand before nodding off.

## Personal Reflection

- How might your initial impression of Carlton's self-described problems impact your treatment plan with him? What was your sense of his motivation to make changes?
- How did Carlton's race and socioeconomic status influence your perception of him as a man?
- What adjustments do you make as a clinician when your client is racially or culturally different than you?
- How does fear and shame play into Carlton's slow-motion suicidal tendencies? How might you assess his self-harm capabilities in the future?

## What Makes Carlton a Good Candidate for Group?

Carlton has some motivation to change, especially given his recent brush with death. He needs the support of others who are also working on themselves. His issues of low self-esteem and a shame-based identity are relatively common among depressed men but are ones that are often the most hidden. Carlton has suffered several major losses in his life, including the death of his father at a young age. Carlton has used drugs and food to avoid touching his grief. His suicidal thoughts and behavior suggests that he feels an emptiness inside that is overlaid by shame about not doing more in his life. As he removes the distractions by getting clean and moderating his eating, it is likely that he will begin to feel the impact of loss in his life. The group might provide Carlton with a safe environment to talk about his inner life with others who will want to hear about it and be ready to help him push through it.

Carlton's ethnic background and childhood experience would bring a diverse and intersecting perspective to the men's group and give him a forum to talk about its effects. Talking about race, prejudice, and socioeconomic status would be a beneficial element for all of the men in the group, especially for those who might feel "less than" on the basis of their upbringing, as well as those insulated by their privileged status.

In group, Carlton's difficulty with shame, impulse control, and meeting long-term goals might be acted out through avoidance of verbalizing his concerns or even absence. On the other hand, his issues around shame and disappointment reflect elements of the struggle endured by many of the guys in the group. Ideally, the group might give Carlton an alternative mirror to see himself. The men in the group wouldn't know him as "Pudge." They would be more likely to see him as a multidimensional individual whose history reflects some of his psychological depth.

## NEIL: CHASING TRUE LOVE

Who doesn't want to believe in true love? I have had my heart broken a time or two when I was young because of my belief in true love. It is such a vulnerable state of mind, putting another person on such a pedestal that you feel as if you could not live without him or her. I recall these intoxicating and often excruciatingly painful feelings, having obsessed about a woman so much that I could painfully sense when her attention was not on me, and it hurt. The intensity of feeling peaks like being high on an ecstatic drug and drops into the low of withdrawal, like a toddler who has lost his parent.

Irvin Yalom (1989) wrote a book about his anointed psychotherapist role as "love's executioner." His position was that "true love" was an illusion based on projection of an ideal onto another. It is not fair to the other person, nor to yourself, to actually build a life around it. Yet, if you have grown up watching Disney movies, it seems that most of the stories involve a young couple finding true love and then living "happily ever after."

I pride myself on having a pretty realistic and grounded view of romantic relationships. Often in my work with troubled couples, we often discuss the disappointments and betrayals of that initial promise of true love. "He doesn't talk to me the way he did." "She doesn't seem remotely interested in making love." "He takes me for granted." "She seems angry a lot and not into doing things together." The tact of exploring unrealistic expectations allows couples to see each other as they are while dismantling and identifying the projections. This is hard work. Many couples are not able to achieve a balanced state of seeing each other as unique individuals who were raised in different families and cultures and who handle stress in their lives in distinctive ways.

Then I have occasionally met individuals who blow away all of my analysis about realistic relationships and seem to be diving headfirst into true love. Thirty-five years into this work, I have seen the gamut of relationship issues from nasty domestic abuse to willful indifference. I can count on one hand those who believe and act on what they believe to be true love, taking the risk to let go of what they have for the promise of something extraordinary. Usually it is not in their marriage but in someone they have encountered on their life journey, someone who stimulates the ecstasy and promise that has been lost in their primary relationship. Others crawl up close to the edge of leaving what they know and retreat back to the safety of their predictable life.

Neil, a 54-year-old Caucasian man, initially called me to talk about a "situation" he was not sure how to handle. "I am feeling edgy and excited at the same time. I am not hungry. I am having trouble sleeping," he had said over the phone. I was intrigued. Often men come with a tangible problem that is a "test" to see how good you are at your job. It is also a low-risk way to get in and out of therapy. Theoretically, he can come for one session, "get fixed," and then get out without cracking open the door to the deeper stuff. I have seen this many times. In fact, when a guy tells me with enthusiasm that I really helped him at the end of one session, there is a fifty-fifty chance that I will see him again. On the other hand, if I have listened, given some good feedback, and engaged him to self-reflect but don't get the high praise, the odds are much greater he will return.

Neil had been to a therapist many years ago with his first wife, Savannah, a beautiful woman much younger than him with whom he had two children. She was not really into the responsibilities of being a mother, nor had she figured out who she was, from how he told the story. When the youngest was 2, Savannah just left one day and didn't return. She had been struggling with addiction to pain medication and alcohol. Savannah had been in and out of rehab before she disappeared. Neil was in the first year of establishing himself as a family practice physician.

Julia, Neil's current partner of 27 years, came into his life during the time of Savannah's sudden departure. She was one of his nurses and filled the void of the abandonment chaos. He confided in Julia, and she helped Neil manage his life. She was the right person in the right place at the right time for a man who was overwhelmed with home and work responsibilities. Julia was 4 years older than Neil and had never been married. She was cute, perky, and practical but not the type that usually attracted Neil. She knew Neil's challenges and was willing to take many of them on. She became the only real mother the kids had in their life.

Sitting in front of me, with a recently clean-shaved head, Neil was edgy. His top button on his shirt was undone, and his tie was yanked out, like someone trying to get a noose off his neck. His eyes darted back and forth as he spoke. It was part agitation, part excitement. I thought to myself that perhaps he was in the manic phase of a bipolar disorder, but there was no indication from his history that this was the case.

## Breaking out of a Mundane Life

At a recent medical conference, Neil went out to dinner with some old medical school friends and their colleagues. He was introduced to Amber, a friend's colleague who worked as a doctor in a medical practice in suburban Kansas City. They sat next to each other. She was blond, 10 years younger than Neil, in great shape, and divorced. The way they connected was significant. Amber got Neil's humor, and vice versa. They laughed and talked. During the 4-day conference, they ended up meeting nightly at the hotel bar, losing track of time, and talking intimately over drinks. While nothing sexual occurred, there was innuendo.

"She is beautiful. I don't think I've ever met someone so amazing. I can look deep into her eyes, and she can meet my intensity," Neil shared dreamily.

"That sounds really powerful." In my mind, I flashed on the psychology conferences I had attended, where everyone is a bit untethered from their everyday lives, open to the novelty of attraction without really knowing who someone is. I had been infatuated like that before. It was fun, but then reality would set in and the life I had created would beckon me back. Neil was resisting the beckoning call of his established life, or so it seemed.

"Yes. I've never experienced this before. It's like we could finish each other's sentences. Just amazing."

"So, you have connected since the conference?" I asked.

"Well, not in person, but by text. We probably text each other eight or nine times a day. If we go more than 3 hours without a text, I can feel myself getting shaky."

At this point, Neil was sounding like a drug addict who has been mainlining Amber texts as if they were crack cocaine. Texting is a fairly recent phenomenon that has added a new dimension to our age of instant communication. I withheld my judgment though, because I was curious about the connection they have. I didn't want to jump to conclusions. I kept wondering how Neil's wife, Julia, fit into this? He hadn't mentioned her as a factor in his consciousness. Where was the good old-fashioned guilt? Or was something else going on? Most guys "in love" are not going to see this as a problem worthy of therapy, but something was not right. Neil could feel it but not identify it.

"Tell me more about what you and Amber talk about." I was curious.

"You know, it is everything from 'have a wonderful day' when I wake up to commentary on politics and to how we each are handling our jobs as physicians. I never thought I'd ever say this, but she feels like someone I have known for a long time."

"Sounds like a kindred spirit. You really are giving each other support," I commented.

"Yes. But it is more than that. I love the way she uses metaphors, and I find myself expressing things in ways that I haven't since a creative writing class in college. I feel like a poet, a Renaissance man. Look at this text." He leaned over and showed me one of the interactions in which he wrote, "Like a blossom in spring, I can feel your opening and I crave to be in that space with you."

"I know this sounds pretty grandiose and cheesy, but it is what I am feeling."

I admit that it did seem dramatic and exaggerated, but who am I to judge the creative impulses of two individuals expressing themselves through writing?

"What does Julia know about all of this?" I assumed this would get to the root of his feeling conflicted. Again, Neil surprised me. He just didn't seem like a man racked with guilt.

"Julia is oblivious. She is so focused on making sure everything is going well with the practice from the business side. She is super busy decorating our house, and then she goes to the gym a lot. Actually I don't interact with her much these days. We would never talk like this."

"What are your thoughts about the fact that the two of you are not saying much to each other?"

"It is quite normal to me. Since the kids left home 10 years ago, we have been operating this way. Like I said, she is really practical and organized. She is a protector of our life. This is her strength. Connecting with the inner me doesn't seem to be a high priority for her. I have been pretty much operating on my own. You know I work pretty long hours, get out for some golf every once in a while, watch some television, but not much else, until recently with Amber."

"So you have been living without much of a deep partner connection with Julia. How about sex?"

"Ha. That has not been happening very much. I think the last time we made love was on a vacation to Hawaii last winter. It feels more like we are business partners than lovers."

As Neil spoke about his marriage, it started to make more sense that he would be "blown away" by a woman who paid attention to him. His relationship with Julia had evolved into a practical, convenient, and safe zone where neither was attentive to the more sensual and intimate elements. It sounded conflict free, but it was barren of the passion and interest of a new, exciting connection.

"Amber is hitting spots that have not been attended to in a long time," I added.

"I guess you could put it that way. I long ago gave up thinking my life could be romantic and passionate. In my first marriage, I fell for a beautiful woman whom I loved with all of my heart. Unfortunately, I learned too late that it was one-sided. I put her on such a pedestal. I did anything and everything to try to make her happy. I love my kids, but I'm still pissed at myself for having gone off the deep end with her. While I was attracted to Julia, and still am, she is not the sexy bombshell Savannah was. There wasn't that passion when Julia and I began our relationship. I told myself I didn't need to go in that direction again. It just made me crazy. Better to be even-keeled, productive, responsible, and emotionally stable. That is what I have cultivated with Julia."

"I wonder if a part of what is making you feel so amped up is that Amber is tapping into the passion you long ago retired. Can you really trust this wonderful but intense feeling when you were burned so badly before?" I asked.

Neil was silent. It wasn't guilt about "cheating" through texting, I realized. His discomfort was some unresolved deeper wound associated with being open and passionate. It seemed to me like an unconscious fear of another betrayal, yet he was attracted to the danger like a moth before a flame. Neil yearned for a romantic connection. Was he protecting himself by going for a woman 1,000 miles away? Was his manic edginess the manifestation of the conflict breaking through his consciousness? Was there even deeper abandonment in early history? Did the marriage he was in have the potential to have passion too, but it had been set up to keep it away? Our session ended with plans to continue the following week. Neil didn't compliment me on the session, so I was pretty sure he would return.

## Addicted to Love?

While I swam laps in the pool, I had fleeting thoughts about Neil's situation. He was living a common middle-age male fantasy. Meet a beautiful, younger woman who was totally into you. Feel understood, accepted, and appreciated. Of course, it involves hot sex that never gets old. It is the woman in the Viagra commercial who looks you in the eyes and lets you know she is ready for all of you. As I snapped myself out of the fantasy, I wondered what I would do if someone broke through my outer wall with passionate interest in me. It certainly would not be so easy to intellectually dismiss it when my whole limbic system was lit up like that. I have been pretty good at remaining oblivious to the signals a woman may be giving me in social situations, maybe as my own protection against facing the conflict.

In our next session, Neil recounted more texts and now a few phone calls with Amber. Since he wasn't sleeping much anyway, he started to leave the house around five a.m. to hit the local gym. Neil described being compelled to lift weights and run on the elliptical trainer to get in better shape.

"It is not relenting. Every time I text or talk to Amber, I get more attracted to her. I heard what you were saying about possible betrayal, and I think you are right."

"What do you mean?" I asked.

"As I get more excited about potentially being with Amber, I am also hearing a faint voice in my head saying, 'Run, Neil, as far as you can away from her.'"

"Like a warning light?"

"Yes. It is like my protection is trying to have a voice, but the dopamine and norepinephrine spewing in my brain are overriding it."

Neil was using his medical knowledge to talk about the power of being in love. The closest thing to it was a heroin or oxycontin rush. Usually, you have to wait until you have habituated to the trigger to even have a chance at resisting. By not having physical contact for a release, or seeing the everyday reality of Amber to make her more human and less goddess-like, Neil's brain continued to fire. I wasn't sure I could actually help him much, except to amplify the warning system and get Neil to try to understand what it was about.

"So, Neil, let's try to focus on the voice in your head that says, 'Be careful. This is dangerous.'"

"I don't know if I can. Intellectually, I get that I have avoided being a romantic so I wouldn't get hurt, but why did I let the wall down now?" he queried.

"What is your answer?"

"You are not going to like this, but I tell myself that Amber is different. She wouldn't do that to me. She knows me so well that I can trust her."

"That is a lot of trust for someone you only have known for five weeks. You have not spent time with her in person." Now I did feel a bit like "love's executioner," but I was trying to tap Neil's resistance to the siren's song.

"You are right, but Amber has showed me what is possible. My mundane, practical life is like driving a Maserati 30 miles an hour. She is encouraging me to be a race car at the Monaco Grand Prix."

"So you want to really put your foot on the pedal and off the brake?" I asked.

"Yes. I think I want you to help me shut down the voice of caution. Racing cars have to go fast. Life is short. I don't want to be trapped by my fear."

Now I was thrown off guard. I make it my job to help individuals achieve their full potential. I write in my online profile to those seeking therapy, *It takes courage and strength to want to improve your life. . . . I will bring passion to our interactions and provide you with honest feedback. I will support you in finding meaning in your struggle and create an open atmosphere where you can look at all of your options as you decide how to take the next steps in your life journey.*

I began to believe that Neil wanted to take his life to another level. I was there to help him nonjudgmentally. But I also needed to give him the honest feedback he deserved. I reminded myself that it was about options and process, not necessarily the solution. Neil's passionate self had been awakened, and he was asking me to help him decide how to respond to it. Privately I pondered whether I too was living too cautiously. I say I want to push my limits, but sometimes I too settle for comfort rather than challenge.

"I hear you, Neil. I will help you achieve your full potential, but I also feel obligated to help you thoroughly explore the deeper aspects of your experience. This includes your history with love and abandonment."

"I've known you less time than I've known Amber, but I trust your judgment on this, Fred. I want more, but I don't want to do it at the expense of everything I have worked toward. Let's keep meeting."

## Fearing Commitment

In our next session, Neil let me know that there was a new development. He did not make eye contact. There were droplets of sweat on his forehead. His voice had a less boisterous tone.

"Amber wants to come visit me out here," Neil finally revealed.

He looked down and went silent. I wasn't sure how to interpret this. This would certainly be a reality check for Neil.

"You don't look thrilled," I commented.

"Initially I was super excited, but it's been a few days since she told me this. Now I'm not so sure."

"What do you mean?"

"This means it's real. She is real, too real. My life could actually be impacted. The warning light we talked about has gone on. I really don't know what to do."

"What did you tell her when she proposed the visit?"

"I said, 'Great,' but ever since then I have been overwhelmed with worry. She has brought it up a few times, and I have changed the subject. I keep hoping she will forget about it, but I know she won't. I am starting to feel bad for leading her on."

"So it feels like the train has left the station and now you want to turn it back," I interpreted.

"Yes. I wasn't prepared for it to go this fast. She is pushing pretty hard to see me."

"Tell me more about her and what you are fearing."

"I know that she was married for a while and got divorced a few years ago. She has a 20-year-old daughter, who lives on the East Coast. She is telling me she wants to check out California, where she can be outside more and not work so hard to have a healthy lifestyle. She also talked about how we would spend more time together and how I would feel about splitting with Julia. Like I said, I am okay with Julia. I don't hate her. We just have a stable, convenient relationship minus the passion. I want the energy and excitement of Amber but none of the reality of what that might mean. I want my stable life and I want a passionate life. That is not possible. Is it?"

So one of the ingredients for true love to succeed is that it has to be stronger than any other relationships. When you are not in a relationship, it is not that difficult to fall for someone promising and attractive. I met my partner on a trip far away from home. I had been single for 3 years after a divorce and had no real role or obligation. She was also available, so the attraction could actually be acted upon. The boundary that made it "safe" was that my home was 1,000 miles away. We could handle the intense intimacy for a week.

A nonhostile, functional 27-year marriage is a pretty solid castle to take down. It is a fortress of predictability, history, and stability, regardless of its faults. An exciting three nights plus two months of texting from 1,000 miles away doesn't quite have the force of a long-established, comfortable relationship. Neil was facing this reality and feeling what it might mean to chase what he believed to be true love. As the session closed, I encouraged him to explore what was beneath his binary choice of "all in" or "all out."

"That must feel like a lot of pressure. What is keeping you from letting her know this is happening too fast for you?" I asked.

"A part of me doesn't want it to end. I am in love with her, and setting limits might break the spell." Neil blushed. "I can't believe I just heard myself say that. I have been so into the texts and calls, but to make it real means my life will have to change."

"Change is actually pretty frightening. You've had a pretty stable life for the last three decades," I reminded him.

"Maybe too stable, but this feels like blowing it up."

"The fear is really talking to you. What happened to the attraction?" I asked.

"It is still there. I can imagine running away with Amber to an island with nothing to distract the two of us. But life isn't like that. The realistic part of me is swooping in on this."

"Before you run from one extreme to the other, why don't we spend the next session talking about you and betrayal. I sense that something is operating below your consciousness that is not letting you see any of this very clearly."

"You are probably right. Neither choice gives me what I want."

Neil cancelled his next session and hesitated committing to another appointment. This was strange. Neil had been so insistent on seeing me. I wondered if the topic of betrayal had triggered a strong avoidance reaction. Maybe the whole conflict was too overwhelming and he was checking out for a while. I thought about giving him a call 3 weeks after our last session, but ultimately I believed he would call back if he wanted to pursue psychotherapy around this. Maybe he had just retreated to his marriage, cut off the Amber communication, and acted as if it never occurred. I moved on, occasionally thinking about Neil and the fantasy. In my mind, I chalked it up to a guy who had come to the edge of his comfort zone and decided to return to what he knew.

## Repeating the Pattern

Eight months later, I heard from Neil. He asked if it would be okay to schedule an appointment that week. He added, "I'm going to bring someone important to the session with me." I was pleasantly surprised to hear from Neil and very curious about whom he might be bringing to his session. It crossed my mind that maybe he was coming with Amber, but that seemed pretty unlikely. My realistic side thought, "He's renewed his relationship with his wife, Julia, and wants to work on his marriage."

Neil had grown a goatee. With him was an attractive woman who had blondish-brown hair and looked to be in her 40s. They sat down together on the couch. Their hands touched. I was fully expecting him to introduce her as Amber.

"It has been a while. I want you to meet Susan." I nodded to her, thrown off. Who was this Susan? What happened to Amber? What happened to Julia? Where is this going?

"Susan and I started our relationship a couple of months ago. But first maybe I should catch you up, Fred. We haven't seen each other in a while."

"That would be helpful, Neil."

As if he could read what I was thinking, he added, "Susan is very cool with who I am. I don't hide anything. I wanted her to be here at our session so she could see how I think and also be open to talking about our situation." I talked to Susan about confidentiality and its exceptions, as well as whether she had ever gone to counseling before, but otherwise waited for Neil to explain.

"Thank you for helping with Amber. After our last session, I had the balls to tell her that it was going too fast. She was pissed. I had not seen that side of her. She called me names and let me know that she didn't respect me. It was so vindictive and cutting that I ended up hanging up the phone. Talk about a spell being broken. She went from siren to witch. All the craziness I had wanted to avoid was on full display."

"How come you didn't try to come back to therapy sooner?" I asked.

"I thought the situation resolved itself. Now I could go back to my normal life and not have to worry about Amber or anything threatening me. I thought you cured me, so no need to return." Neil smiled.

"Until now?" I asked.

"Yes, until now. So, I think I may have been fooling myself, and I want your help to get a reality check."

I was pretty disoriented with Susan in the room. Neil was acting as if she was not there, yet she was there. He was saying he would bare his soul in front of her. But I didn't know her. I hoped she would begin to say something so I could grasp the dynamic in the room.

"I will try to help, but Susan, what is your connection to all of this?" Before she could respond, Neil interrupted.

"Susan and I have actually known each other for many years. She has been our local drug rep. We have always been really friendly. It went to another level a couple of months ago." He smiled and looked over at Susan, who broke into a forced smile. I detected some discomfort with her being in this intimate environment with me. I was not sure she had bargained for this.

"Neil and I ended up having dinner together as a part of our rep meeting. He and I shared about our marriages. We had so much in common in relation to our spouses and the lack of passion. Something electric happened as we talked. By the end of the evening, we were the last two in the restaurant. It was pretty magical."

This sounded almost like the same story Neil had told me about Amber. The difference was that this was close to home. Both lived in town. There wasn't 1,000 miles separating fantasy from reality. I was confused. How was this going to work?

"I think I know what you are going to say, Fred. You are going to ask me about my fears. My fear of abandonment. My fear of betrayal. My fear of messing up my life."

"So, yes. What about those fears?" I asked.

Neil looked over at Susan. She nodded to him, as if she were giving permission.

"We have both decided to leave our marriages. We are going to do it together at the same time. We thought you could help us strategize and get through it. You know, the emotional part."

I was dumbfounded. These two conspirators had found in each other the strength to make the move they couldn't make alone, together. Neither had been able to pull the trigger by themselves. Both must have been ready. They seemed to have no idea about how this might work out. I knew it would not get any easier, only more complex and intertwined. Yet here they were in front of me, seeking guidance and maybe approval. They certainly seemed to believe that true love would save the day.

I saw Neil and Susan for four sessions. Despite my attempts to help them reflect internally on their actions, they focused on the practicalities. How do we tell our partners? What about our kids? How much should we see each other before we let others know? How should we handle lawyers and separation/divorce agreements? In reality, they didn't need me for this. What they wanted was someone in authority to witness their actions, who would not judge them for falling in love with each other. That was me. As if on cue, I was dismissed as their therapist once the plan was hatched and acted on, left to think on my own about true love and its ability to exist in the real world.

At a fundraising dinner in town at the end of the year, I caught a glimpse of Neil from the other side of the room as he walked from the bar with two drinks in his hand. His shaved head was gone. His hair had grown back, leaving a prominent bald spot. He was much heavier than when I had last seen him. With my eyes, I followed him back to his table. He passed the extra drink to a woman I didn't recognize. She smiled at him. He laughed and touched her arm. I imagined her as his newest incarnation of Savannah, Amber, or Susan.

Neil caught me glancing at him and came over. "Dr. R., good to see you. I would like to come back to therapy. I know this isn't the right venue, but I think I could use some help."

"Neil. Give me a call next week and we can set something up," I replied casually, knowing that his follow-through behavior would be the real indication if he was being polite at the dinner or really wanted to work on himself.

### Personal Reflection

- How do you feel about passion in intimate relationships? Can the passionate aspect of a marriage be rekindled? Does it need to be for a marriage to survive?
- Do you have any countertransference issues with Neil and his situation? How might you use your judgments or projections to understand Neil's relationship pattern? How do you channel your passion?
- How might you confront Neil's tendency to leave treatment once his conflicts became less intense? What might you want to focus on upon his return?

### What Makes Neil a Good Candidate for Group?

Neil seemed to have idealized the potential for women to fill the intimacy void in his life. Although I suspect there was unspoken abandonment in his childhood, Neil seemed to latch on to women with whom he could fantasize a merging. His long-term relationship with his second wife broke the pattern. It made him feel as if he were a boy being taken care of, rather than a man chasing a romantic love. The series of affairs seemed to play out in a similar way each time—infatuation and then retreat when the relationship became more real. He was stuck in a relationship pattern of merger and escape, one that he avoided confronting in his therapy.

Neil's conflict with women seems to tap a universal dilemma for many heterosexual men. He has teetered between shutting himself down and acting out his sexual desires. The mundaneness of a businesslike marriage was acceptable until he was exposed to unexpressed passion that occurred in a relatively safe environment away from home. Neil could use the feedback from other men to explore his inner life. Although it might be uncomfortable for him initially to be a part of an all-male group, with no women to seduce or please, Neil might potentially become more comfortable with himself as a man in this type of environment.

On the other hand, Neil's tendency to avoid conflict and his lack of insight might make him a high risk to drop out of a group that presses for intimacy. His Casanova-like dating behavior has superficially reinforced his masculine identity while keeping him from reflecting deeply about his relationship patterns. His presence in the group might spark discussions and conflicting concerns about intimacy, passion, and the unintended impact of abandonment among the members. Ideally, he might be confronted on his avoidance behavior and be encouraged to be more authentic in his self-understanding.

# 8

# The Body Talks

The mind and body are so intimately connected that disturbance in one area often affects the other (Brower, 2006). Physical pain can lead to feeling depressed, but emotional pain can also manifest itself as a physical symptom. In this chapter, you will meet two men who are struggling with pain in their bodies. Lee, a former athlete, lives in constant pain that seems to worsen when he experiences psychological conflict. Ray, who has lived a bohemian lifestyle, confronts a diagnosis of cancer, which requires him to reflect on the meaning of his life. Through psychotherapy both men learn to interpret the body's signals as important data about the psychological aspects of their lives.

## LEE: MASKING CHRONIC PAIN

Pain and aging seem to go together. I know that when I have activities, visits, and events to look forward to, I am more likely to lose track of my age. However, if I am hurting physically, I am very much reminded of my chronological years on the planet and impending mortality. Experiencing pain takes one's attention away from the pleasure and possibilities of the present and future. Pain can override everything. It is a constant reminder that something is wrong. The brain is stuck in a mode of sending and resending a warning signal. That is not a pleasant way to live. Chronic pain is highly correlated with

http://dx.doi.org/10.1037/0000132-009
*Deepening Group Psychotherapy With Men: Stories and Insights for the Journey*, by F. E. Rabinowitz

a depressive outlook in life and a leading contributor to addictive behavior and negative thinking (Trivedi, 2004). It is one of the reasons that many individuals consult physicians and sometimes psychologists.

Lee's partner, Rona, had made the initial call to inquire about whether I had openings. Although normally I feel that this is a sign of a codependent relationship, I could sense her frustration and desire to help her husband find a way to deal with his depression. I encouraged her to have him call me to set up the appointment. Two days later, Lee contacted me. As we talked on the phone, our conversation got pretty deep quickly.

## Facing Depression

"I guess my wife talked to you about me and my negativity. She means well. I can be a real pain in the ass," Lee started.

"Sounded like she really cares about you," I replied.

"Yes. She keeps me going. Not sure I would be here without her."

"You mean here talking to me or here in life?" I asked, sensing some deeper meaning in his comment.

"Ha. You picked up on that. Good question. I guess both. I have thought a few times about just driving my car off the road or wish someone would just finish me off. I couldn't do it, though." In my experience, this passivity toward death is a sign of depression, or maybe it's just an acceptance of the inevitability of death we all face. In my life, things have to be pretty bad for me to think about a passive death, like not waking up from sleep. Most of the time I fool myself into believing how important it is to be here. I set goals, write lists, and have activities in which I can invest myself. This can often ward off the existential truth that we are here temporarily.

"Either way, you don't sound excited by life," I responded.

"You got that right. While I have you on the phone, Dr., do you think it is possible to change who you are at my age?" This was a very poignant question. It is at the core of the work I do. If I believed it wasn't possible, I couldn't do the work. I decided to be diplomatic and hear what Lee thought. I also had no idea how old Lee was.

"If you are asking me if it is possible, I would say yes. But at the same time, I would say that most of us get pretty comfortable with who we are, even if it isn't working very well," I replied.

"That sounds like me. I can imagine that I could change, but my track record doesn't bode well for that happening. I've made many a New Year's resolution that I didn't follow through on."

"I hear you. It's your call if you want to give counseling a shot. It certainly won't work if you don't want to try."

"You know, it would be much worse for me if I didn't try. My wife would be even more on my case, and who knows, maybe an old dog can learn something new."

Lee, an African American man with a very athletic build, met me in the waiting area. He was 6 foot 4, muscular in his arms and legs, with a slight paunch. To me, he looked much younger than his 55 years, maybe mid-40s. Lee was dark skinned; had a shaved head and a goatee; and wore a basketball T-shirt, shorts, and sandals. I was most surprised by his contagious smile. You would not look at this man and say that he was depressed. I was reminded again of how well most men hide their pain. Lee could have been on the cover of the AARP magazine as a poster boy for health, yet here he was in my office. This was the same man who expressed suicidal ideation and not much of a will to live.

As Lee walked into my office, he nodded to me and immediately noticed the punching bag hanging in the corner.

"I guess boxing is in bounds in this office," he joked.

"Yes. I do have some gloves in case you want to take a few swings."

Lee laughed, then grimaced. He braced himself as he sat down on the sofa. He slowly lowered himself and moved around to get comfortable.

"Injury?" I asked.

"How about injuries? I have trouble sitting anywhere for more than a few minutes. Is it okay if I get up and walk around when I need to?" Lee's physical movements told me a lot about him. It was obvious he was in pain. This belied his superficial healthy appearance. I wanted to know more.

"Sure. Tell me about your injuries."

"Where should I start? It has been a long road."

## Sports and Identity

Lee used the recounting of his injuries as a way to tell me his story. He had grown up in a tight African American community in south Los Angeles. His described his dad as a "mega-athlete" who played high school and college basketball. Lee and his three brothers were encouraged to make sports an important part of their lives. As the youngest, Lee reaped the benefit of his brothers' experiences. He was included at a young age in their games, giving him an advantage against his peers in sports like football and basketball. Lee was a high school All-American in football, getting a scholarship to a major Division I college, where he played running back.

"Yes. I thought I was God's gift to the world in high school. I set a football rushing record for our high school and was the leading scorer on the basketball team. What I didn't realize was the toll all that took on me."

"You mean physically?"

"Physically and psychologically. During my 3 years playing varsity football in high school, I must have run the ball 500 times. You take a lot of hits. At the time I thought I was pretty invulnerable, but by my senior year, I started feeling a bit beat-up. Back then they didn't have concussion protocols like they do now. I'm sure I suffered some pretty major concussions and just kept on playing."

"What about the psychological part?"

"You know, I think I believed I was indestructible, like nothing could go wrong. I would say to myself, 'Be cool. It is all going to work out.' I did not listen to the voice that said, 'Watch out' or the voice I hear nowadays that says, 'So what, big shot.'"

"Can you say more about those voices?" I asked.

"I thought I would jinx myself if I let in any negative thoughts. So I actively suppressed my own doubts and stayed away from anyone who was going to be critical of me, including my dad and some of my coaches who tried to remind me that I could still improve. But as a 17-year-old who led the league in rushing, I thought I knew better."

"So you were a cocky 17-year-old who had the proof of his worth on the football field. What were you like off the field?"

Lee grimaced again and pushed himself up. He stood up and rubbed the lower part of his back.

"What was the question?" he asked.

"You look like you are in a lot of pain," I said, distracted by his discomfort.

"Yes. It is not easy to sit. I have some damaged vertebrae in my lower back. I also have some permanent nerve damage in my neck. Each of my knees has had three arthroscopic surgeries to repair ligaments."

Lee lost his focus several more times during the session. As it came to a close, I asked him how it was to share with me some of his life experience.

"I wish I could tell you it was great, but in reality, my pain began to take most of my attention. It was hard to sit here after about thirty minutes."

"What if we schedule our meeting for a half hour instead of an hour? Do you think that might help you focus?" I asked.

"You know, that may not be such a bad idea."

### Exploring Beneath the Mask

We scheduled our next meeting for the following week. Now that I knew Lee's story, I was more sensitive to the subtle sadness in his face. He wore a similar outfit, which I realize was mainly for comfort. He again sat down gingerly.

"You know, Dr. Fred, I did think about our meeting from last time this week. I feel like I might have sounded too prideful about my past. You know there are a thousand athletes with stories like mine. I am not that special. I naively thought I was going to end up in the pros and geared my life around doing that. I wish I had studied more in college and actually graduated. Not many people know that I never finished my degree. I just took courses I thought I could pass based on recommendations from teammates. When my eligibility was up, I was done with school. Without football, I didn't see the point. The only good thing was that a few of the guys on the team actually were pretty good at business. They got me in on the ground level of a sports marketing company and that has been my salvation in terms of earning a decent salary and still being connected to sports."

"You seem a bit remorseful about not finishing the college degree."

"It's another secret that I keep from people. Everyone sees me as the upbeat ex-athlete who knows how to make good marketing deals. No one really knows any of the stuff I've told you."

"What if they did know about the you beneath the surface?" I queried.

"It is hard for me to imagine that scenario. I hope I am not being disrespectful, but you seem like an intelligent psychologist, but you are also a White man. I have noticed all of my White friends don't seem to carry around that extra suit of armor I have to as a Black man. You know, they are cool people, but I can't imagine they know what it's like to be seen with suspicion wherever you go. I have to make people feel comfortable so they won't see me that way."

"Like a false surface personality?" I asked.

"Yes. Like that. If you were just a colleague or superficial friend, you would see me as laid-back, nonjudgmental, like nothing really bothers me."

"But that isn't necessarily what you think and feel inside," I commented.

"No. As you can tell, I'm a bit of an ass. I do judge. My wife is the only one who I let see this side of me. . . . And now you."

"How does that feel to let me see this part of you?" I asked.

"You know, I guess it is your job . . . the confidentiality and all. I believe you want to help me, so the only way that is going to work is for me to be up front with you."

"I appreciate the trust. You keep saying you are an ass, but honestly I haven't heard anything like that in here. What is it that makes you feel like an ass?" I asked.

Lee smiled. Then it turned to a grimace. He put one hand on his lower back and steadied himself with the other. Lee seemed to drift off.

"I don't know what to say. I can't remember what you asked me. My back is really acting up. I think I need to move. It's probably almost time to leave anyway. I'll catch you next week, Dr. Fred."

## Confronting the Psychological Pain

Like a running back who had found a hole, Lee was out the door after 20 minutes in session. He moved pretty well for a guy in pain and started me thinking about how he had left the first two meetings. Both times, I had asked him to go a bit deeper with comments he had made. The pain came right then. I wondered whether it was conscious. I knew I would have to bring this up next time, but not in a way that would activate more defensiveness. Even though I knew his pain was real, it also seemed to have become a way for Lee to get out of difficult situations.

When I saw Lee again, he seemed a little less upbeat, or maybe I imagined that because I knew some of the pain underneath his mask. He again sat carefully down, looked up at me, and asked me if I could review what we had talked about in the first two sessions.

"My memory has been a little spotty. I know that I was very open with you about some of my past, but I keep feeling like there is something I can't recall about our interactions. It is bugging me."

The opening was there for me to bring up his avoidance of deeper material. I had thought about what I might say, but I was still very aware that I didn't want to make something an issue that wasn't. Two times is not enough of a sample to say this is a pattern.

"Lee, you know, what was clear to me was how much pain you carry with you. Twice I asked you about the more psychological pieces of your pain, and both times the physical pain became unbearable and you didn't answer. I wonder if it is uncomfortable to talk about yourself, especially when it doesn't fit with how you want to see yourself?" I wondered whether this interpretation would hit.

"You know, you may have something there. I didn't realize that my pain acted up right when I was about to talk about something personal. What was it I didn't say?"

"In the first meeting it had to do with how you saw yourself off the field, and the next time it had to do with being an 'ass' and letting me see this part of you that no one else sees except your wife," I replied.

Lee looked down, squirmed in the chair, and then caught himself.

"Oh yeah. You know, I started to notice my back throbbing when you were talking just now. Are you saying that maybe I focus on physical pain as a way not to face my psychological pain?" he asked, genuinely inquisitive.

"What do you think? Why might you not want to face the psychological pain?"

"Doesn't make a lot of sense to me. I am here to talk about my psychological self. I have a medical doctor to talk pain to. Weird. But I have been stuck for a long time, so I am not saying you are wrong, just I don't get it."

"All of us develop coping mechanisms or defenses to reduce psychological stress. I wonder if you somehow used your physicality to cope with difficult emotions?" I was stretching here, but Lee seemed open to exploring the mystery of his avoidance behavior.

"Interesting you say this, Dr. Fred. Since I can remember, I have used playing sports as a way to cope with everything. If my parents were fighting or if I had too much homework, or if I didn't know how to handle a situation, I immediately went outside to play a game. Everyone knew me in junior high as the guy who carried a football around with him, even to class. I laughed about it and liked the attention, but I never really even thought about why I was doing it. So you are saying that the reason I can't figure stuff out about myself is that I always blocked out the negative emotions by distracting myself physically?"

"In your body, does that fit as an explanation for you?" I asked, wanting him to feel it, not just intellectualize about it.

"You mean, does my body have some sort of response to what I shared?" he asked.

"Yes. Do you notice anything? Maybe your breathing, heart rate?"

Lee smiled. "Wow. I do feel something right here." He pointed to the area below his chest. "Are you saying that my body is talking to me, Dr. Fred? I hear that saying all the time, but it feels kind of crazy."

"Well, yes. Your body talks to you all the time. Your sensitivity to the pain you feel is your body signaling you, but it can also talk to you about psychological and emotional issues as well," I added.

"So in beating up my body through sports, the intense pain I feel is its main voice. I'm used to that, but I don't really know how to interpret all the other signals it's sending. Fascinating."

"What is your body saying to you right now?" I asked.

"I feel kind of excited. I can feel my face, like a smile, but more global."

"Yes. You got it. You said 'fascinating,' which is like a way of interpreting this new information you are more consciously aware of. Psychologists call it 'insight.'"

Lee did not mention his pain as our 30-minute session came to a close, but he still walked carefully out of the office, obviously in some pain but not as much in the forefront of his consciousness.

Over the weekend, I headed up to the local mountains to go skiing, one of my winter passions. It had been brisk, but the snow was pretty good for Southern California skiing. I had probably made 15 runs, hadn't fallen down, but when I got into my car to drive home, I could feel my lower back seize up some. I wedged myself into my car, and by the time I got home, I was in excruciating pain. I asked my wife to give me an ice pack and tried to numb it. By the next morning, I could not get out of bed. Just moving pierced me with extreme discomfort. I developed sciatica in my leg so that walking felt almost impossible. As I lay in bed with an ice pack on my lower back, I reflected on Lee's condition with extreme empathy. I tried to bargain my way out of it. I told myself I just needed to rest for a day, but over the weekend the condition seemed to get worse.

As Monday rolled around, I could not walk without wincing in extreme pain. I felt like a 100-year-old man. The intensity was so debilitating I cancelled my college class and called my clients to reschedule. I could not remember ever having had so much pain. I got an appointment with my doctor and chiropractor, hoping this would be temporary, but I was deluding myself. By Wednesday I was on a regular dose of over-the-counter pain relievers and prescribed muscle relaxers. It was enough for me to move slowly to my car and to shuffle around. The one good part of this horrible pain was that my empathy toward others with disabilities was off the charts. I began to notice people who walked with a limp, or who had a cane, or seemed to be having trouble with any kind of movement. My pain was putting me in touch with a part of humanity that I had either ignored or barely acknowledged.

When Lee walked in for his appointment, I stayed in my chair. I was wearing an ice pack under my pants. I had worked hard on staying focused on my patients rather than myself, but it was difficult to override the throbbing in my back and the sciatica shooting jolts. Like an athlete who had been injured and wanted to stay in the game, I tried to gut it out.

Lee saw me grimace as I reached up to shake his hand.

"Dr. Fred, what's wrong?" He immediately recognized the appearance of extreme pain.

"Just some back pain," I minimized.

"Looks pretty nasty. Is that a lower back, pinched nerve? Those can be excruciating."

"Yes. You know it. I tweaked it over the weekend, and it is not getting much better."

"Hate to break the news to you, Dr. Fred, but the tenderness of a herniated disc can last for a while. I've had a couple in my day."

"Thanks for the support, I think." I tried to get out with a smile.

"You probably been icing and heating it off and on. You taking the muscle relaxers?" The tables were turned. He was the doctor, having a good dose of empathy for me.

"Yes. I have been trying. You know, Lee, I understand better your desire not to talk about pain too much. It makes me focus on it, and I am doing everything I can to focus on what I have to do."

"Dr. Fred, I believe you have entered my everyday zone. It's not so easy to stay with your feelings and thoughts when the pain is taking all of your energy," he said.

"So, how are you doing?" I asked, deflecting my own pain to try to focus on his.

"I thought about our last meeting, and it was like a lightbulb going off. It made me rethink much of my life as a boy and man growing up. I realized that my struggles were self-inflicted," he reported.

"In what ways?" I asked.

"You know, the whole being-an-athlete thing was just a natural way for me to find structure. My dad taught me about competition and that everything was like a game. So rather than listen to my body, I made my body into something that would help me win and compete. Nothing wrong with that, except that maybe all of life isn't about competition. Why would I need to be competitive with my wife? Why would I want to compete with my own kids? I guess I got stuck and it cost me."

"How?" I asked.

"Well, if my model is always to compete and win, I check out when that's not happening. I noticed this week how much I tuned out Rona when she spoke to me in a pretty caring way. I had to fight to keep myself present with her. I so bad wanted to go watch TV or find something else to do."

"Wow. That is incredibly insightful, Lee. How did it work for you?"

"I noticed, but I am not sure I said anything that made her feel any better. I did realize that she is trying to help me, not bitch at me. Sometimes I felt like saying, leave me alone, but most of the time she was really trying to connect."

"Where in your body did you know that?" I asked, reinforcing Lee's newfound way of hearing himself.

"You know. I watched her face and saw it in her eyes. I almost cried. My eyes got watery when she was trying to help me," Lee said in reverie, as if he was replaying the interaction in his mind.

For a moment I forgot my own pain as I listened to Lee's description of a change in how he was receiving his world. He made a lot of sense. I noticed the time, and our session was almost up. Lee looked at me, and I could feel his eye contact. I felt his warmth and compassion. As if on cue, he said, "Dr. Fred, I think it is time for me to go, but I am worried about you. Keep rotating the ice and heat. See you next time."

### Personal Reflection

- What was your reaction to Lee's presenting concerns? How might you have handled his acknowledgment of pain in the sessions?
- Do you believe that Lee's identity as an athlete impacted his coping with life situations? What about his identity as a Black man? How might this have kept him from asking for help sooner?
- What were your thoughts about the therapist's physical pain becoming a part of therapy? How might it have helped or stymied Lee's progress in coping with his own pain?

### What Makes Lee a Good Candidate for Group?

Lee has isolated himself from other men, although there are many men who perceive him as a friend. Very few know of Lee's struggles with not only pain but also the impact of subtle racism on his life. He often feels as if he has to be better than or appear less threatening because of his ethnicity. On top of that, he struggles with chronic pain. Lee's sense of invincibility was shattered with his injuries. It took him from being an optimist about his future to a person who had trouble seeing a positive scenario. His pain represents vulnerability, a constant reminder of his mortality. Although he is good at masking his underlying depression from others, this pain provides a portal toward his deeper self.

In the group, Lee might have trouble trusting the other members, given his history. He might hide behind his traditional masculine mask of the ex-athlete, but the group could also become a safe place for him to be himself without the front. The group could benefit from Lee's sharing his inner thoughts and feelings and could know him more intimately than just through his appearance or athletic prowess. Lee has the potential to expand his repertoire as a man by being in a group that values authenticity over appearance and the sharing of emotions over hiding them.

## RAY: LIFE AND DEATH

Ray, a White man with grayish-blond hair flowing over his shoulders, floated into our session in a worn, blue Grateful Dead T-shirt; jeans; and sandals. He had a big grin, making it hard to imagine him not having just smoked a little weed before entering the room. I smiled back, recognizing pieces of myself embodied in Ray's presenting persona. Ray and I initially met at a Dark Star

Orchestra concert. This tribute Grateful Dead band has served as the top "minor league" talent squad for the later incarnations of the Dead following the 1995 death of lead guitar player Jerry Garcia. Our encounter at the break between sets of the concert brought a deep discussion about the meaning of life. Toward the end of our spontaneous talk, he asked about what I did. I told him I was a psychology professor and psychologist who specialized in working with men. I ended up giving Ray my professional card before the show resumed and thought nothing of it.

It was now 3 years later. Ray had kept my card and contacted me. He wanted to talk through a few things and thought I might be a good person with whom to do this. I was at once flattered but also a little uncomfortable. I had met Ray under nontherapeutic conditions, and now we were converting it to a counseling relationship. I wasn't sure how this was going to work, but I liked Ray and trusted myself to figure it out as we went. If it was going to be more of a friendship, I would take it in that direction, but if it was truly a man asking me for professional guidance, I would need to better define the boundaries of our relationship.

Ray did reek a bit of marijuana, but I did not jump to any conclusions. I wanted to hear his story. I knew it must be significant for Ray to be contacting me 3 years after meeting me by chance at a concert.

"So good to see you, man," Ray began. His big smile automatically put one on my face. What could this happy hippie possibly need from me?

"You too, Ray. What brings you to my world?" I asked.

"I still remember that DSO concert a few years back. The conversation we had stayed with me. I thought, I should probably go see that guy Fred. It was intuitive, but I wasn't sure why at the time."

"What was it that we talked about that stayed with you?" I asked, genuinely wondering what I might have said that had that kind of impact. I hoped that I had not said something profound while he was under the influence of some hallucinogenic drug, but it was possible.

"You seemed to have a pretty grounded perspective on life. I recall you telling me that living in the present was akin to being fully alive. Getting stuck in the past or future was what created anxiety. You said, 'Right now is what we have to make our lives what we want them to be.'"

I was impressed that he took that from our interaction. I did recall the intensity at the time, but I know I've probably said it before in class, too. It's a common humanistic existential axiom of committing oneself to be "all in" with current behavior and interactions.

"I'm glad that was a powerful memory that you could access," I said.

"Well, I wouldn't be here if I didn't have a dilemma. You were the one I thought of when I was contemplating who to talk to about it," Ray continued.

"Before you let me know, Ray, I need to get some clarification. Are you consulting me as a professional therapist?" I asked.

"As opposed to what?" he asked.

"As opposed to me just being a friend whose opinion you are asking."

"What is the difference?" he asked.

"Well, if you are talking to me in my professional role, then I want you to know the benefits and limitations. I have ethical responsibilities, and we will need to discuss payment, et cetera." It felt strange to have to go through the professional boundary talk with Ray, but it seemed like he was more comfortable with me leaving it ambiguous.

"Oh. I assumed I was talking to you in your professional role. Sorry if I implied otherwise. I have been to a therapist before and know about the rules." I felt relieved and ready to engage. I do believe that Ray was about to tell me something important, and I interrupted him. I hoped he would continue where we left off.

## A Life-Threatening Fear

"So, go ahead, Ray. You were about to let me know about your dilemma."

"Yes. I am having a harder time than I used to being able to live in the present. I am afraid that I have become more of a worrier than a dreamer."

"What do you mean, Ray?"

"Fred, I have always been a free spirit. I've traveled all across this country. I have lived in communes. I have lived in Iceland. I have been a 'Deadhead' who followed the band for a couple of years. I have always been comfortable with the road and trusting I would be provided for somehow. My current job involves traveling for a software company. I make decent money, but . . ." Ray looked down. A trace of a tear rolled down his cheek from his watery eyes. I waited for a minute.

"What is it, Ray?" I asked, sensitive to the unexpressed emotion.

"I had been having some problems with my stomach . . . you know, keeping down food. I've lost some weight. I was hesitant to go to a traditional doctor because of some of my experiences. That's a long story. My dad was a physician, and he and I never agreed on the role of Western medicine. Anyway, I avoided consulting a 'real' doctor and ended up medicating myself using pot to enhance my appetite and maybe cure whatever was messing up my stomach."

"How has that worked?" I asked. I thought of my own struggle with Celiac disease, which has made me very careful about what I eat. It is a disease of the small intestines, so I had some empathy for types of stomach problems.

"I guess it works as a way for me to mask the symptoms. I have still been losing weight," he continued.

"How long has this been going on?" I asked.

"About two years. I just kept smoking weed, which has become a pretty normal state of mind for me. I'm used to functioning on it in my everyday world, but I know it's probably not that great. A couple of weeks ago, I finally went to a real medical doctor, a gastroenterologist, who ran some tests on me. That is why I came to you. It turns out I have stage 2 colon cancer. Luckily it hasn't spread to other organs yet. There, I said it. I have not wanted to deal with this, but it is always on my mind. I am scared." The color had drained from his face.

"Talk to me about your fear, Ray."

"You know, I am the same age that Jerry Garcia was when he died—54. I know I am at the mercy of the universe, and when it's my time, it's my time, but I haven't been able to accept it. I want to."

"That sounds like what you say to the fear. What is the fear saying to you?" I asked.

"Scared shitless, as Crosby, Stills, Nash, and Young said at Woodstock. You know, I thought I was comfortable with death. I have always run close to the edge, but this one I didn't see coming. I have choices to make. People to tell."

"Even though none of us get out of this life alive, it is hard to be comfortable with death," I responded.

## Marijuana as a Coping Mechanism

"Do you mind if I use my vape pen?" asked Ray, showing me the smokeless new device for tobacco and cannabis. Given the circumstances, I was faced with another ethical dilemma. It's like a client having a beer during the session. I knew he had smoked before he came in the session, but doing it during the session? I could see some faceless judge letting me know my license to practice would be taken away for unethical behavior in session.

"I know this is hard, but maybe see if you can hang in here without getting high," I replied, setting the boundary.

"Man, I told you I smoke this stuff to help me with my stomach pain. I have a medical marijuana card. I thought you'd be cool, given our Grateful Dead background."

"Ray, you can do whatever you want. I am here to help you with the emotional part of this. From that perspective, it seems like the pot is going to dull not only physical pain but also the emotional pain."

"I know, but I am pretty desperate. I'll be right back." Ray walked out of the consulting room to go outside to vape, I assumed. I was not comfortable with his smoking in the middle of the session, but I also did not want to abandon him as he opened up about his cancer. I think he went out of the room to be respectful of me. Again, I am not sure clients need to worry about the therapist's needs, but in this case he was also taking care of his own needs.

When Ray returned, he seemed more relaxed, and there was a renewed scent of marijuana.

"Sorry, Fred. I know that smoking in a session isn't cool, but I am pretty torn up and it does the job temporarily," Ray said, eyes downcast, suggesting some shame at his dependence.

"Look, Ray, I want to be helpful. Seems to me like you are scared but also wanting to approach the cancer treatment with some courage. I can be here while you talk out loud whatever comes into your mind and whatever emotions are stirred up."

"I know that. I just may not be as ready as I thought," he said, looking down at the floor.

"We are near the end of the hour. Do you want to schedule another time?" I asked.

Ray hesitated. "Let me get back to you on that." He then rambled toward the door before looking back at me. "This has been pretty intense. I need to absorb it a bit."

"I understand. Call anytime."

I really didn't expect to hear from Ray again. He had taken his shot at talking to a psychologist. When we got close to the issues, the fear and anxiety became too intense. The marijuana seemed to be doing the trick in terms of short-term relief, but the more existential concerns were rumbling in his soul. He had some big decisions to make around treatment, as well as how he wanted to handle the cancer emotionally.

## Facing Death Anxiety

It was about one month later that I got a call from Ray, saying he was more ready to face some of the deeper issues. This time, when he took his seat, I was aware of not catching any whiff of weed. Ray wore a black, silhouetted Garcia shirt with the late guitar player's beard prominent.

"Decided I am ready to make some progress, Fred. I am not willing to live in denial limbo land anymore," Ray said with conviction.

"What changed, Ray?" I asked.

"That scene in your office around my weed consumption was pretty eye-opening. I realized that I was just getting foggier and more chickenshit. It wasn't helping. I was more pathetic. The other thing that happened was I got a notice from Esalen in the mail and saw a workshop called 'Facing Your Fears.' I remembered that we had talked about Esalen, the retreat place in Big Sur, at the show. You told me you had run some workshops there, and I had gone back in the '90s to a meditation retreat. I was still on the mailing list. I headed up there last week. It was great timing for what I needed to work on."

"I'd love to hear about it, Ray. What was it like for you?"

"I went there with the intention of facing my death anxiety. I know there is a chance that this cancer is going to kill me before I am ready. I wanted to be in a space where I could voice it. You know how beautiful the place is, set on the cliffs above the Pacific Ocean. Just walking around the grounds made me calmer, like I was a part of the world, not just some isolated being."

"I know how calming and therapeutic it is being in an environment like that."

"Yes. Being able to also interact with other souls who are struggling openly made it easier for me to open up. I had some emotionally intense talks in our group and in the tubs that overlook the ocean." I fondly envisioned the hot springs built into the side of the cliffs that allowed for whale watching by day and stars by night. The waves crashing on the rocks below dominated the soundtrack of Esalen.

"Tell me about your experience sharing your fear."

"The workshop was led by an older couple, who seemed wise beyond their years. The woman named Rising Hawk had obviously done a lot of inner work and seemed to emit light and warmth. The guy, Raimey, had long white hair. He looked liked Gandalf from *Lord of the Rings*. He had a gentle spirit but carried some higher level awareness about dimensions beyond the earthly one. It felt like I had the soulful parents I never really had. The others in the group were very open and welcoming as well. I felt like I had this deep, rich family for the week."

"It does sound like a really nurturing space. Was there anything in particular that changed your approach to more directly facing your cancer?"

"It's funny you say that. Toward the end of the week, I had this very intense event. You know I am a music fanatic, but one of the guys in the group was a didgeridoo player. The sound that came out of that thing was otherworldly. It was like something the Dead might do during an instrumental part of one of their songs. The sound was low and melodic, but definitely not Western. On the last day we were doing a guided imagery around traveling inside of ourselves for some kind of wisdom about how to handle fear."

"Sounds interesting."

"As I shut my eyes, the sound seemed to summon up spirits inside of me. It was like the most vivid dream I had ever had. I saw these animated Native American people with face paint floating around me, dancing and chanting. I knew that Esalen was built on an old Indian cemetery. It was like the spirits from the dead were making themselves visible to me. Physically, I felt like I was flying like a bird, dropping into the darkness of underground cliffs. I started weeping uncontrollably. Tears were running down my face while my eyes were still shut. The longer the didgeridoo sound came, the more I wept. But it felt like hopeful tears. I sensed that there might be another dimension to our reality. Death on this plain of existence might not mean total death but rather a transformation to another dimension. In fact, as I am recounting this, I can feel the tears starting to come into my eyes."

I listened and felt goosebumps on my skin. I recalled a dream I had about death that had a similar feel. Ray seemed authentically moved.

"The crying must have felt relieving. You had been holding a lot of emotion around your fear," I said.

"Yes. The release and the vision made me less afraid. I am ready to face the unknown. Instead of it feeling like an execution, it is feeling more like a transformative event. I am here to talk out with you all of the pieces of this. I need to not only decide about treatment, but I also need to figure out how to handle my family, including my daughter."

"We have a lot to catch up on."

### Confronting the Unfinished

Ray and I spent the next several sessions talking about how he wanted to live his life, given the cancer. We also spent time exploring his earlier life and the relationships he had with his parents and siblings. It was hard for Ray to face some of the unresolved issues around his estranged wife and his daughter.

"I feel pretty guilty about how the marriage disintegrated and how it affected Marianne, my daughter."

"Say more about that, Ray."

"Alisa, my ex-wife, and I were not very good communicators. We met at a Dead show when I was 24. She was only 18. Alisa had run away from her family. They had been emotionally abusive to her, and she was smoking a lot of weed and couldn't wait to get away. We ended up standing next to each other, smoking and dancing. Our bodies seemed to get to know each other before our heads did."

"What do you mean?" I asked.

"You know. We were touching, and she ended up coming back to my van after the show. We made love and just held each other, like two people who needed extreme comfort and merger. The beginning was just like a dream. We followed the Dead. She made art that we sold in the little village that sprung up in each parking lot the Dead were playing in. We bartered with other Deadheads for food and pot and the other necessities. It also led us to live in our first commune together with some of the folks following the band."

"Sounds like it was idyllic for a while."

"It was great until it became crazy. Alisa and I started to drift apart, since we were actually pretty different intellectually. I had gone to UCLA, studied philosophy and creative writing. She had dropped out of school at 16. The remnants of her abuse were never far away. Sometimes she would just take off for a few days without any warning or communication. I figured she needed space, but later I found out that she was pursuing some other relationships and doing some harder drugs. Our run lasted about three years. Marianne was conceived when we were in the last phases of our relationship. It was messy."

"What ended up happening?"

"I stayed around for the birth, but Alisa took off with the baby. Another long story, but to cut to the chase, she ended up living with some guy up in Oregon and they raised Marianne. I was relieved to get out of the whole mess. I ended up going overseas. I worked for a few years in Iceland as a bartender in an American hostel and pub."

"So you got away, but right now you said you are feeling like things are unresolved with your daughter?" I asked.

"You know I have a long story about this. She and I didn't see each other for the first 10 years of her life. She finally tracked me down. We met and made a good connection, but of course it was weird because she was growing up in rural Oregon and I was living down here in California. We made a promise to each other to try to do two visits a year, but this was not taking into account her mom or stepfather's wishes. In the end, I talked with Alisa to allow us to get together for a week in the summer each year. When Marianne turned 18, she went on the road like her mother had. I didn't hear from her for 3 years. We have had a relationship of sorts over the past 6 years. She lives up in Alaska with her boyfriend. We communicate through email and Facebook but have only had a couple of live interactions in this time."

"Sounds complicated."

"I really do care for her, and I am trying to figure out what I really want from her as I do battle with the cancer."

"What do you want?" I asked Ray directly.

"I really don't want to heavy her out. I want to protect her, but I also am feeling like she should know and decide for herself how involved she wants to be."

"I hear you trying to protect her, but what is it that you want from her?"

"Honestly, I just want some love and maybe share more of myself with her. I'm not sure how she sees me. Maybe she represents my legacy?"

"Your legacy?"

"Yes. She will live on, and I worry that I will be nothing more than some absentee father figure who will never be mentioned to her own kids. Selfishly, I want to feel like my spirit will live on, and she is the only one who can do this in a physical way."

Ray shook his head and then stared off, not making eye contact. His last statement hit home. The incompleteness of his relationship with his daughter, the lost time, words not said, and the emotions not shared were overwhelming. He wept, a stream of tears running down his face. The bohemian life he had led allowed for freedom but also left him a bit empty in terms of closeness and connection. After several minutes, he turned to me.

"Fred, do I seem like a monster to you? Am I that bad of a father? Is this the consequence of my avoidance all these years? This is probably the pain I didn't want to feel."

"You are confronting it now. That counts," I countered to his self-hate.

"There is a lot there. Beyond Marianne, there are my parents, whom I have kept at an arm's distance too. I want to reconnect with them. I have a lot of catching up to do with them too."

"I'm ready to support you in that, Ray. Let's spend some time in our next few sessions exploring all that you need to say."

Ray and I met twice a week for the next 3 weeks going over his life history in more depth. Ray started chemo and radiation treatments, coming to sessions even when he was feeling like crap. I was impressed with his work. With death staring him in the face, he was on a mission to close the gap on the unfinished business of his life. Ray contacted his daughter and let her know of his condition. She told him she was going to come for a visit. As the time got closer, Ray asked me if he could have her come to our sessions. "I want to be able to talk to my daughter like I talk to you. It would be great if she would come here, and then maybe it would jump-start us talking more deeply to each other." I agreed, as long as he let his daughter know ahead of time and let her make the choice to come or not.

Ray, now completely bald from his radiation treatments, was dressed in a *Dark Side of the Moon* T-shirt when he next came to meet with me. His blue eyes matched those of his daughter, Marianne. She also had his nose and smile. She had long brown hair and a nose ring, and she wore a skimpy tank top with her tight jeans. Marianne had a laid-back demeanor, given she was here for a therapy session with her dad. Ray and I had done some rehearsing of possible dialog and scenarios, but I was curious to see how this would play out live. I took the lead to structure the session, but I really put it into Ray's court.

"Marianne. Good to meet you. Your dad and I have been working together. If you have questions, please feel free to ask. Otherwise, I am here to help or guide if needed. Ray?" Ray was on the edge of his seat but seemed ready for the encounter.

"Marianne, I wish I could have talked with you without needing a therapist present, but this is who I am. I want to connect with you, and I don't trust myself alone."

"Ray, I mean Dad . . . I guess you are right. That felt a little weird to call you Dad. I'm glad you let me know about what was happening. I was scared that I'd come down and see you lying in some bed wasted away. You look pretty good for someone who is battling cancer."

"I think that is a compliment," Ray responded with a smile. Marianne had some of Ray's wit and humor. "Hon. I am sorry for not keeping better track of our relationship. I have been a bit in my own world."

"It goes both ways, Dad. I have been doing my own thing for a long time. I have never felt satisfied with standing still. I have been on the move," said Marianne.

"I guess we are not that different, Marianne, in our longing to be on a journey. But we have been on different journeys. I wanted to approach you here with a request. I want to know about your life, and I want you to know about mine. As my pal and psychologist, Fred has said to me several times, it is not that easy to just ask someone to open her life to you. I know we need to spend some time, do things together, and build a relationship that can allow for deeper sharing."

"Dad, I am a little taken back. I want to connect, but I am far away from being open. The years growing up with Mom and my stepdad feel very real, and I don't know how to let you in on that. The years since have been lots of wrong turns, wishing there was someone who really had my back." Marianne's eyes got watery as she spoke. Ray looked directly at Marianne, held her hand, and said, "I wish I could have been there. I want to hear about everything. I will also answer any questions you have about me that you wondered about." They hugged each other for a while without words.

Ray and Marianne left that day having started a process of reuniting. Marianne moved down to this area to live with her dad as he went through his treatments. Ray continued to meet weekly with me as he embraced the unknown.

### Personal Reflection

- What ethical concerns might you have in the way that Ray entered therapy? What was your reaction to his desire to smoke pot in the session?

- What are your thoughts about Ray's lifestyle? What are your reactions to the changes he experienced when he went to the Esalen retreat to face his fear of death?
- What were the most significant consequences of Ray facing his own death? How do you feel about Ray trying to make up for lost time with his daughter and using therapy as a means to share more intimately?

### What Makes Ray a Good Candidate for Group?

The rift that Ray had with his father, a traditional physician who had little time, seemed to be the start of his seeking alternative ways of getting his needs met. The separation from his wife and child and his rejection of mainstream culture left Ray vulnerable to feelings of abandonment, which he found ways to deflect. The cancer diagnosis had the most impact in exposing his fear but also provided Ray with a conduit to his deeper self, a rich tapestry of emotions and relational longing.

Ray has a social orientation and seems to thrive in interactions with others. He moved around as young man and still has a job where he travels. Ray's drug use and lifestyle did value "hanging out," and the substances may have added a creative and peaceful atmosphere for interpersonal relating. On the other hand, the drugs also distorted reality and led to blind spots in self-awareness and direction.

The men's group would be a way for him to share more intimate parts of himself and get support. His issues around keeping others at a distance from his internal process would be challenged by the other men, who would spot his defensive style. Although Ray might be tempted to avoid depth, he would bring a social and articulate openness to the conversations in the group. Others struggling with loss, regret, and feelings of mortality would also resonate with his story and self-expression. Ultimately, Ray could really use the support of other men as he battles cancer and tries to reconnect with the family he left behind.

# 9

# Dealing With Loss

Men often downplay the impact of loss in their lives. Male gender role socialization discourages men from crying and sharing their grief with others (Cochran & Rabinowitz, 1996). This socialization can create conflict for men who are feeling deep sadness and are ashamed of being able to express it fully. In this chapter, you will meet two men who have been impacted by significant losses in their lives. Justin has grown up without a father and is dealing with his mother's cancer diagnosis and the recent death of his mentor. Michael has sustained multiple losses, including the death of his mother, his wife leaving him, and his dismissal from his administrative position. Psychotherapy leads to acknowledging the losses and having permission to grieve.

## JUSTIN: THE POKER PLAYER

Ambushed by the colored lights and the ambient noise of falling coins from slot machines, I walked steadily toward the poker room unfazed. Like Odysseus hearing the Sirens' song, most people find the slot machines irresistible. I do not. I may be fooling myself. There is a big difference between pure chance and having to engage in a skill to get lucky. Poker is perfect for those of us who believe you can make your luck rather than be its passive recipient. Although fate might be destined, we have the ability to maneuver toward it. With the power of observation and pattern recognition, one can influence the

http://dx.doi.org/10.1037/0000132-010
*Deepening Group Psychotherapy With Men: Stories and Insights for the Journey,*
by F. E. Rabinowitz

outcome of a game, even with its random cards. By keeping track of people's tendencies, I can read their reactions and use this data to influence my behavior.

For a psychologist, no-limit hold'em is as close as I can get to applying my training for financial and psychological advantage. That may sound selfish, but I spend most of my days as a therapist, professor, and human being helping others through those reads. Hold'em is my chance to use it for myself. I have found it healthy to have outlets where I get my needs met. It makes me a better therapist and provides me with empathy into the lives of those with whom I work. Poker is a game of power, and in this world, it is naive to think that we are not constantly engaged in power struggles with those around us for resources, recognition, and love.

It was Tuesday night, and all of the regulars were there to play in a Texas Hold'em poker tournament. Poker is the perfect capitalist game, where the person who ends up with all of the chips is the winner. Each hand gives you a chance to outplay others, who get the same distribution of cards you do over time. I love tournaments because they are fair. Everyone buys in for the same amount of money and starts with the same number of chips. It is a game of survival. You need to accumulate chips but also not lose them. Once you are out of chips, you are gone. It rewards both patience and aggression, a balance that encourages risk taking but also caution.

Every time I enter the poker room, I feel the adrenaline rush through my body. It is part fear, but also anticipation. As I handed Randy my money, he asked me, "Feeling lucky tonight, Fred?" I said what I always say: "Hope so." He handed me a randomized ticket that had my seat position and table draw. I know that this random seat draw may give me a spot where I get wonderful cards or, in my worst fantasy, the crappiest hands possible. Who knows who will sit next to me? Will they be good players, lucky players, fun players, or obnoxious players? Tonight I was assigned to Seat 1, next to the dealer at Table 4. With the time clock ticking down, the players with their tickets found their assigned seats. It crossed my mind to do this with my college classroom at the beginning of class. Maybe students wouldn't get so comfortable always sitting in the same spot.

I automatically studied the players, most of whom are men. Because I have been a therapist for men, this is second nature to me. I assume that everyone is a little anxious starting out, so I notice how people control their nerves. Some are quiet, others talkative, and some just edgy. They shuffle their chips. A few wear hats and clothing designed to intimidate or entice. Men outnumber women 9:1 at most 10-handed tables, making women more noticed. Often they take advantage of this situation by dressing provocatively or flirting, just to throw off the concentration of some of the older, traditional men at the table.

As the dealer began to throw out the cards, I took a deep breath and anticipated the two cards he would deal me facedown. In Texas Hold'em everyone gets two cards, which are known only to the player and no one else. There is a round of betting, during which you can bet the minimum, fold your cards, or raise the bet. The players sort themselves out by communicating to the rest of the table the perceived quality of their hands. The dealer then spreads out three flop cards that are visible to all players. The idea of the game is to make the best hand with your personal hole cards and the community cards. After the flop, the betting continues, with the players jockeying to portray a strong hand or fold. This happens again with a fourth faceup card, called the turn. Finally, a fifth card, the river, revealed, which allows for a final round of betting. Each hand plays out this way.

Sometimes someone portrays a great hand, and the rest of the players fold before the dealer lays out the rest of the cards, so you don't always see the winning hand. This is the basis for bluffing, as no one really knows what the other player has unless he or she has to show it at the end.

When I am in poker mode, I seek to take advantage of all the information available, from the betting patterns to facial expressions. After folding several hands, I peeled one card up, and it was the ace of hearts. Whenever I get an ace, I hope that the other card is a picture—Jack, Queen, King—and in the best-case scenario another ace, the strongest starting hand in poker. Oh my. . . . It was the ace of spades. I trembled inside and hoped that I had not given away the strength of my hand.

### Playing Poker Against My Client

Across from me was a young man I knew very well. He was in his late 20s, wore a Los Angeles Dodgers baseball hat and mirrored sunglasses, and exposed only a flat facial expression. With deliberation, he said "raise" and put out a large bet. The other players seemed intimidated by him. There were folds around the table, until it reached me. Normally this was a no-brainer. I could re-raise to announce that I have a "monster" or just call the raise to disguise the strength of my hand. I hesitated.

The young man across from me was not just some random poker player I could intimidate. He was Justin, one of my clients in my practice. We had nodded and made eye contact earlier, but now we were in a game he knew better than I did. Not only did I know he played poker for his livelihood, I had knowledge about what lies behind the mirrored shades. I knew it would be possible that the two of us would cross paths in the poker world, but up to this point it hadn't ever occurred. As I sat across from him, I was a competitor, not his psychologist, but still I paused. My professional training that led me to helping others with emotional support and psychological insight was in direct conflict with the point of this game—to take advantage of the other players' vulnerability. I didn't ever recall this scenario coming up in my grad school ethics class. I reflected on our relationship.

Justin was the only child of a single mom, Jeanna. She worked as a waitress at two different restaurants, bringing in enough money for them to live in an apartment in a poor neighborhood. Justin's father did send money but lived in another state and made occasional "guest" appearances. His dad showed up at his 11th birthday party one year, and he came to Justin's high school graduation. He never stayed long enough for Justin to get a read on who he was. In the past, Justin had been suspended from school for cursing at one of his male teachers and had been fired from some fast-food jobs by male bosses.

Although he was a marginal student, mainly because he was on his own most of the time at home, Justin excelled at math. He took to numbers, statistics, and even algebra without much need for assistance. Eventually Justin became an apprentice to an older electrician, Mario, who could see Justin's potential. The electrician taught Justin everything he could, and in exchange Justin was more than eager to do the tough, physical parts of the job that his boss was not capable of performing.

I peeked again at my aces, also called pocket rockets and the weapons of mass destruction. I looked up at Justin, who stared at me with his flat-faced disguise. Time slowed down as I pondered my bet. I caught a glimpse of the kelly green felt, the playing field for our game. Justin started to finger and flutter his chips rhythmically, waiting for me to act. I wondered if he was thinking about me as his psychologist, or was I just a competitor he was getting ready to take down?

I recalled Justin telling me that he got his poker start after work, with Mario guiding his initial foray. Mario taught him at the cheap cash table how to read players and do the calculations on his odds for winning. At home, Justin found the websites partypoker and Full Tilt, which allowed him to play lots of hands for small stakes. When Justin won his first online tournament, he was hooked. An initial investment of $30 turned into $50,000 over the next 3 years. Although initially skeptical, Justin's mom became a huge fan and supported his play. Much of his earnings went back to his mom so that she could live in a better place in a classier neighborhood.

Mario, who seemed to care less about electricity and more about poker, supported Justin's game and invested in him to play in live tournaments. With his online play, cash games at the local casino, and bigger buy-in tournaments, Justin was able to go full-time at poker. For a while, he moved to Las Vegas, but he returned home when Mario, who had decided to retire, asked Justin to take over the electrical business. Justin continued playing poker locally and online, and he ultimately sold the electrical business, returning a nice chunk of money to Mario for his retirement.

Just when it seemed that he was achieving financial and career success, disaster struck. Mario suffered a fatal heart attack. Within a month of Mario's death, Jeanna was diagnosed with Stage 4 breast cancer and given a poor prognosis. This is when Justin found me, referred by a friend whom I had helped.

## Loss and Pain Open the Door to Therapy

I realized as I sat across from him at the table that I knew his pain. I knew the losses he had endured, and yet in the moment he was stoic and steely.

I admired his strength. It is hard for most men to come to a therapist under any conditions. Justin had to be a tough guy to protect himself out in the world. Although he could be himself at home, the environments he inhabited—school, work, and poker—were not places for showing any kind of weakness. Being perceived as a momma's boy results in a quick learning curve in elementary school for most young men. If you did not want to get beat up or be made fun of, you kept your emotions to yourself. In his work world, there was a lot of posturing and storytelling that avoided the doubts and worries most men have under the surface of their lives. In poker, weakness was exploited.

In the office, Justin and I initially bullshitted about poker a bit. I recognized his Full Tilt hat and asked him about his hold'em experience. This conversation helped him feel as if he was talking to somebody who might understand him. When we got to his real reason for being here, he hesitated.

"It's my mom. She's in bad shape. I am not handling it very well."

"What do you mean, not handling it well?" I asked.

My directness seemed to force him to move toward a more honest appraisal. "I can't sleep. I can't concentrate. It is hard for me to care about playing poker, and that's how I make my living."

I nodded. He tried to keep a straight face, but his eyes started to water. A single drop rolled down his cheek. "Sorry. I didn't want to be emotional," he uttered as he fumbled with his sunglasses. I could see that he was tempted to put them on indoors.

"It's okay. She is important to you," I replied.

"Beside my business partner, she is the only one who has been there for me. I can't imagine her not there. I can't see the future."

"What do you mean, you can't see the future?" I asked.

"I've always imagined that my mom would be a part of my life. I set goals, but she is always a part of the picture. I don't know what it would be like to be without her."

In contrast to the poker face that confronted me in the casino, Justin's uncovered eyes closed, his face contorted, and then he sobbed. I watched him from my chair a few feet away. It didn't feel right to say anything. He had been holding this in, and now in my office he was letting it out. I tried to grasp the depth of his pain. As a clinician, my job is to have empathy while maintaining my own sense of self. It is not always easy. Often the molten lava of emotion under the surface needs to be released. Although women have been socialized to accept tears, most men have not. Justin had learned not to share much of his pain. His mother had enough to worry about, and he could be a good listener.

"It sucks," I said after what seemed to be a long silence. I avoided the typical therapist trap of trying to get at male feelings too quickly. Too much exposure could make this a "one and done" session. "Sucks" uses the language that men are used to and takes away some of the shame associated with feeling sad and weak. He responded.

"You're telling me. On top of finding out about my mom's condition, the only older guy I ever trusted just died last month. It has been terrible. Mario saved my life when I was lost. He taught me how to be a man, how to work in the world, and got me into poker."

### Using Poker as a Way to Explore Deeper Issues

Justin saw me regularly. Usually we eased into our sessions with poker stories, before diving into the deeper waters. During our early sessions, Justin shared with me how he had been living his life, with a focus on how he could best be there for his mom as she underwent chemotherapy. He was the diligent son, taking her to appointments, cooking, cleaning, and being her caretaker. His anxiety and depression, although still present as fears, were less inhibiting.

"The doctor said her probability of full recovery was 20 to 25 percent after the mastectomy and chemo. That gives us a chance."

"It's like any two cards against a pair," I said.

"I wish it was better than that. But you know, Mom has been talking a lot more to me about her life. She's been telling me stuff I never knew about my grandparents, her sister, and even my dad. I sense she is not afraid to die."

"How is her lack of fear impacting you?" I asked.

"You know, when I first started seeing you, I would have done anything to save her. Now I still want her to come out of this healthy but am less fearful of the future."

"What's different?" I asked.

"This may sound stupid, but I realize that life is like a long poker tournament. You try to stay alive by playing smart and getting yourself into high percentage situations. But even then, you don't have control over everything. Pocket aces get cracked 20 percent of the time, even though that is the best starting hand."

"Yes. You can only do as much as you can, but some of it is really not in your hands. What did you find out about your mom that you didn't know?"

"I found out why she and my dad split. I just thought he was an asshole who didn't care about us. She told me that they weren't ever really together. They had met at a camp as counselors one summer when they were both about 18. They fooled around some, had sex one night, and Mom ended up pregnant. It wasn't until after the camp ended that she knew. She told me she didn't want to tell him because she didn't want to screw up his life. He was going to college and had dreams of being a doctor."

"So she didn't tell him about the pregnancy?"

"No. She ended up looking him up when I was about 5 years old. Turns out he was in medical school on the East Coast. She sent him an e-mail about me. He wrote back, felt really bad, but was already engaged to someone else. Instead, he sent her money to help with raising me."

"Wow. That is a very different picture than you assumed all these years."

"Yes. I actually would be interested in knowing him as a person someday."

"Someday?" I queried.

"Not sure I can take it on right now. In my head I want to do it, but there is something in me that really doesn't want to know."

"What do you think it is?" I asked.

"I've carried around so much anger at him over the years. It's not so easy to just be 'it's okay.'"

This is not uncommon for a man to sit with years of accumulated resentment in his body that he can't let go. In my earlier years as a therapist, I received training in bioenergetics. This therapy integrates the mind and body by helping an individual release psychological tension through a physical outlet, which can then be discussed with the therapist. I threw Justin an old tennis racquet I keep for this type of situation.

"Go ahead and slam that thing on the couch cushion."

"What? You want me to hit it?" he asked, confused.

"Yes. Just see what happens. I am trying to help you with that feeling you say gets in the way of wanting to see your dad."

Justin started cautiously but soon was pounding with more intensity.

"As you hit, say whatever comes to mind in relation to your dad."

Justin stopped. "You want me to talk to him as I hit it?"

"Yes. Trust me. I know you have intellectually changed how you view him, but you are still carrying around a lot of anger."

He continued pounding and the words started to come, and then were spoken in rhythm with the racquet contact.

"Where were you? Why didn't you come and see me? Fuck you! I don't care who you are. I don't care about you. Go to hell!"

"That's what you are really feeling. No wonder it's hard to forgive him," I commented.

"I want to, but it has been too many years of hating his guts, acting like I don't care."

"With the intensity of the emotion you just showed, I think you do care."

"Damn. I wish I didn't care. I have always secretly wished he'd show up to live with us, but I told myself to forget that happening."

"I think it's going to take some time to talk about all of what you have 'secretly' held in before being okay with getting to know him. You might even be able to tell him how you have felt."

"I don't want to meet him this angry. I do want to catch him up on my life, but right now I think I'd rip into him."

## Encountering the Missing Father

Over the next several meetings, Justin and I talked about his fantasies about his dad, both positive and negative. As his father figure in therapy, I was the object of some of his rage. I expected this would happen, as it involved wondering if he could really trust me, or if I too would abandon him. The primitive level of his emotions surprised him. At the end of the session, he would apologize for being angry, not wanting me to recapitulate the father abandonment scenario that had dominated his life. One of the most interesting strings of discussion came to his fascination with poker and how it might relate to his rage.

"You know, I think one of the reasons I love 'live' poker is that I really like to mess with the older guys."

"What do you mean?"

"I know a lot of them play conservatively, so it feels satisfying to play like a 'wild man' against them. They can't figure out whether I am playing them for fools or if I am just that good." Justin smiled. It was a dark satisfaction for him. I understood it. I think a part of why I enjoy poker is because I also find it satisfying to be aggressive with people I would normally be nice to.

"That makes sense, Justin. You do get to channel some of your anger at those older men. Do you think this connects to your anger at your dad?"

Justin grinned again. It was as if I were having a conversation with his shadow.

I sat with my pocket aces, facing Justin. I was in his domain right now. This was his professional world. I was the amateur. We sized each other up. He gave me a sinister smile. He knew me as his therapist and mentor, but did he know me as the poker player?

"Re-raise," I announced, looking directly at Justin.

The smile on Justin's face got bigger. "Aces, Doctor?" he said out loud to the table as he peered at me through his mirrored sunglasses.

I didn't say anything, but he knew. I probably gave off some tell that let him intuit that I had a big hand. He continued the stare. I could feel him studying me like I studied him in therapy. His scan was unnerving. I broke eye contact and looked down. He knew now. He figured I wouldn't raise him with anything other than aces. His cards left his hand and landed faceup. Kings!

"Show me the Aces, Doc. I fold."

I obeyed his command and turned them over. We both grinned, as if this had been predetermined. Although I would later get knocked out, I did watch Justin amass a large stack of chips. He made the final table. I was envious. As I began to move toward the exit, I caught Justin's eye and nodded. He saw me and got up from the table and shook my hand. "Good run, Doc. See you tomorrow at your place. Got to be able to pay your fees, you know."

I felt his warmth. "Take down the tournament, Justin. Let me know how it goes."

"Will do, Doc."

## Personal Reflection

- What is your reaction to meeting Justin at the poker tournament outside the therapy space? How might you be able to anticipate this obvious dual relationship? What makes this unique encounter potentially therapeutic?
- How does Jason's transference with the therapist help him move closer to working through his issues around father loss? How does exploring his multiple losses help Justin understand his anti-authority tendencies?

- How do you feel about exploring your own issues around being a helper? How might competitive games allow for balance in the life of a therapist?

### What Makes Justin a Good Candidate for Group?

Loss and potential loss are the wounds that made Justin reflect more about his emotional depth. It was not until his mother's cancer appeared that Justin seemed to experience the cascading effects of a lifetime of losses, including his father and male mentor, Mario. These losses gave Justin an opportunity to realize the impact of loss on his life and how he had been coping over the years. Growing up without a father and having to rely on a mother who was usually at work pushed Justin toward autonomy and resulted in a significant conflict around dependence. Although he may have needed nurturing, Justin was successful in navigating a world that reward independence and toughness. His work reinforced his stand-alone style, yet he also sought male mentors to guide him on his path.

The presence of mainly older men in the group really gives Justin an opportunity to be supported and mentored. He might be hesitant to make himself vulnerable initially, given his strong traditional masculine self-structure. I can imagine that he would also challenge other members with his more overtly masculine approach to confront their underlying assumptions about their coping and defense systems. As a younger man, he might also elicit projections from the other men of themselves earlier in their lives, as well as potential father–son dialogues. Given Justin's underlying losses, the group might form an emotional container for him, a space to express his anger and sadness in a way he hadn't before.

## MICHAEL: THE SCIENTIST

Having both intelligence and a scientific outlook can be a blessing. One can analyze, dissect, and understand the world. It might also have an unseen downside. With a highly logical approach to life, there is a tendency to use this over other forms of knowing oneself. It is not uncommon for the rational intellectual to use prowess as a way to distance himself or herself from an emotional life, which often is not as neat and understandable. My experiences in academia have informed me that to be incredibly smart is not equal to being happy. In fact, intelligence run amok can also lead to difficult dilemmas in relationships and life outside one's field of study.

Michael, a university science professor and administrator, contacted me in early January through my website. He said he was looking for a clinician who had the "academic credentials" to work with someone with his background. My site shows that I am a licensed clinical psychologist as well as an author of books and articles and a tenured professor. This seemed extremely important to Michael, as he did not want some "half-baked therapist, who wasn't steeped in theory, research, and practice." I just listened. I implicitly understood that this was the way that Michael felt as if he wasn't wasting his time. By making sure he was in the company of highly educated individuals who could think rationally, he could protect himself and guarantee that he could display his strengths as a highly educated person.

"I never perceived myself as needing any kind of assistance, so I want you to know that although I may speak freely, I am not really comfortable with this arrangement," Michael started out in his first session. The formality seemed forced. Michael was dressed in a blue suit with a yellow tie. He had a pale complexion, was clean-shaven, had thinning gray hair, and wore wire-rimmed glasses. It was not hard to notice that his belly gut looked out of proportion to his other body dimensions. Michael's eyes darted suspiciously as he spoke. I noticed that he had an American last name, but from his facial features I guessed he had some East Asian heritage. Something about him made me feel sad. I sensed that he had dealt with a lot of pain and was using his skills as a scientist and administrator to keep himself busy and distracted. To slow down to deal with the tumult inside seemed threatening and would take skill on my part to tease out.

"I understand. What is it that you want to get from talking to me?" I asked.

"Good question. Let me consult my list on my phone," he responded, pulling out his smartphone and scrolling to his list of issues.

"Here are my top concerns. Number 1, I am not happy, and I want to figure out why so I can enjoy my life. Number 2, I have lost my joy, my purpose. When I first started in grad school and academia, I was so motivated to publish, to become more. Now I often dread getting up and going to work. Number 3, I am struggling in my primary relationship. No passion. Nothing. Not horrible, but I question why I am still in it."

"Those are big issues," I replied.

"Yes. I wouldn't be here otherwise. I am hoping you can shed some insight on why I am not thriving. Objectively, I should be fully enjoying my life. I have a good career, I have published some important papers, and am devoting myself to the university as a dean. There must be a confounding variable, something I cannot identify."

"Tell me a little bit about your life story. It would help me to have some context for your concerns," I replied.

I needed a foothold to connect with him. Michael spoke in paragraphs that distanced him from his inner emotions. What he described was depression, and this was one of my fields of specialty. Having worked for much of my adult life in academia, including more than 10 years in administration, I understood the kind of pressures present in this environment. I also knew many faculty members, both their public personas and some of their private tribulations. Academia was competitive, was often petty, and involved highly intelligent individuals clashing around faculty governance, work conditions, and the treatment of students. Given his demeanor, I found it hard to imagine Michael functioning comfortably as an administrator. He had the aura of a scientist, not the approachability of someone adept at working with people.

"I've never done this before. Are we going to need to talk about my childhood? I don't quite see the relevance of wandering through events from ages ago."

"It is possible that some early patterns might have been established at a young age. It would certainly help me to understand you if you told me a bit about your upbringing. Please share with me anything you deem relevant," I countered, noticing I was "upping" my vocabulary to match his. Michael took a moment to respond. His head tilted right as if he was trying to capture some ancient video from his mind's eye.

## Achievement Doesn't Lead to Happiness

"I am an only child, adopted as an infant, who grew up in an academic household in upstate New York. My parents were in their early 40s when I was brought into their lives. My dad was a mathematics professor and my mom a chemistry professor at Cornell. They met at the school where they both taught early in their careers."

"What do you recall about your childhood with them?" I asked. Again he took a moment to access memory.

"I don't recall too much. You know I am 52 years old. That was a long time ago. I recall that it was pretty quiet in the house. Both of my parents were introverted, like me. They liked it that way so they could think. We used to go up to Lake George for a couple weeks each summer, but my most vivid memory is both of them reading books out on those Adirondack chairs. During most of the academic year, they worked and I went to school. I graduated top of my class from high school."

"That is impressive. You said you didn't have any siblings, but what about relationships with friends or extended family?" I asked, wondering how isolated Michael really was.

"What about them? I don't recall having too many close friends. . . . At least no one I have kept in touch with beyond high school. I was pretty nerdy. I studied a lot and spent most of my free time reading books. I was really into science fiction. I think that influenced my desire to go into the sciences and do something that related to space travel."

"So you spent a lot of time alone with yourself and your books."

"Yes. My parents were always reading or working, and I found my solace in reading books. It felt like a family activity we did together, a perfect introvert space. I guess you could say I was destined for an academic life."

"Hobbies or other activities beside reading?" I asked, curious about this type of upbringing.

"I took piano lessons and would spend time learning classical pieces. It was challenging and a bit of a change-up from reading. Other than that, I wasn't much of a social person." I listened and nodded.

"Tell me about your experiences beyond high school."

"I ended up going to college at Cornell, where my parents taught. I studied physics and history, double majored. Then I went to graduate school out of state and got my doctorate in physics. Got my first position out west at one of the elite schools for scientific research. The rest is history. About five years ago, I decided I wanted a new challenge, so I applied and was chosen to be the dean for one of our graduate programs."

"That is pretty impressive trajectory. I am sure there was much more to the journey," I injected.

"Of course. I published some really good work in particle physics and was a member of a science team that worked on one of the space missions," he recited without much emotion. In terms of accomplishment, Michael was near the top. Somehow that was not enough to bring him the joy in life he had hoped for. I wondered how much space he had created between his intellectual pursuits and his emotional life.

"You had said to me earlier that you weren't happy and that you had lost meaning in your work, despite your success."

"That is why I am here. I don't get what happened. When I describe it to you, I should be proud and fulfilled." Michael looked down. I noticed his eyes had watered up, but no tears. "But I'm not. In fact, I am really sad, and I don't understand."

Michael's stoic demeanor now had a leak. I pictured him as he might have been as a young boy rather than a middle-aged man. I felt my own pain in his moist eyes. I reached into my own loneliness, my own journey in academia, and the amount of self-denial it took to achieve. For that moment I could grasp the depth of his grief, yet I didn't have words to describe it. I sat with Michael for a while in silence, not knowing how long he had held down that deep sadness.

"I don't have words for my sadness. I don't feel like I can control when it comes. I find myself crying without reason. That scares me," Michael finally whispered.

"The tears suggest powerful emotion. Have you ever felt this kind of emotional flow before?" I asked.

"Not so out of control. I did recall feeling something like this when my dad died 5 years ago, but it made sense. I lost my dad. I could connect the dots. Humans feel sadness when someone close dies. This doesn't make obvious sense."

"Five years ago was also when you became a dean. Any connection with your dad's death?" I asked.

"I never really put the two together. I believe that was purely correlational. Are you suggesting that I might have made the administrative move in response to my loss?"

"It's possible. I sense you are looking for a rational answer to your sadness. It may be more complex than *X* plus *Y* equals *Z*," I responded.

"I assume that it is. You have worked a long time in your field, published papers and books on depression. Have you seen this before? Is it fixable?" he asked.

## Figuring Out Sadness

I was caught flat-footed by his comments. I had hypotheses but not answers. I did not necessarily see the tears as a negative, but perhaps a signal from some deeper part of him trying to break through the steel computer of his mind. He seemed to have no clue as to what might be flooding him with overwhelming sadness. Rather than answer his questions, I wanted to see where his own exploration might take him. I could help with that process.

"I am not ready to venture guesses at this, but I do want to hear what you have been saying to yourself when these spells happen. How have you been making sense of the sadness and tears?"

"I cannot come up with any rational explanation, so I assume it is something occurring in what Freud might say is my unconscious mind. So given that, I feel inept to tackle the problem. By definition, I can't know what I can't see," he said dispassionately.

"Let's assume that it is something unconscious. Typically, the unconscious is a storehouse of all kinds of data that are not necessarily needed in everyday reality. Much of what we perceive and experience is not directly relevant to our current tasks. For you, the study of particle physics, really does not require much unconscious processing, except perhaps as a way to problem solve. You see data and then have to infer what is going on," I expounded.

"What do you mean?" he asked.

"Well. If you are struggling with a problem, you might not immediately see the solution, so your mind must pull from various neuronal connections to past learning, reading, experiments, and previous problem solving to come up with a novel solution," I explained in my best neuropsychological jargon.

"Yes. That process I get. Sometimes I take naps, and some piece of the puzzle might come into my mind that helps me with difficult problems. Are you saying that process might also be useful with my mysterious crying episodes?"

"Yes, I am saying that. Especially since you are having trouble with rational explanations for your emotions. Are you open to a little exercise?"

"Sure, if you think it will help." Michael had an inquisitive look. His head tilted up, and his eyes widened.

"Please sit back in your chair and close your eyes," I instructed. He relaxed into the swiveled rocking chair. He loosened the top button on his shirt.

"I want you to try to relax your neck and shoulders. Just imagine them becoming less tense. Your mind is very powerful and can actually give a signal to these muscles to loosen up. You might also notice your breathing and take a deep breath and exhale. Let's do that again." I went through his body with him, giving his instructions to relax muscles and to stay attuned to his physical self. He was very compliant and seemed to welcome my direction. As our time was running short, I encouraged him to enjoy the relaxed state, and when I brought him back from the exercise, I asked him about his experience.

"That felt good. Is this something I can practice myself?"

"Of course. That would be a good exercise for you to practice this week before our next meeting. Find some time each day and take about 20 minutes to go through and become aware of your muscles, and work on mentally relaxing." He seemed to leave the office with some hope, given the slight spring in his step as he left the room.

In our next session, Michael again appeared in a suit but had already taken off his tie and undone the top button of his shirt.

"I did the exercise each evening before bed. It made it much easier to sleep. I also felt more relaxed overall this week. Maybe that was the trick."

## Symptom Relief and Avoidance of Deeper Issues

Michael's spontaneous flight into health did not surprise me. As often happens, the act of going for help and finding some technique to change one's conscious reality is a powerful placebo. The immediate gratification and the fact that the tears did not come made it seem like magic. I was skeptical that this exercise would be enough in itself. In fact, my thought was to use it as his vehicle into his unconscious mind. If he could put himself into a relaxed state, he might be less defensive about mining the fragments of his internal process. Maybe this popular relaxation method with its origins in the late 19th century could produce some data he might consider legitimate.

"Tell me more about the practice, Michael."

"Well, I found a time to do it each evening, and it seemed to just calm me. No crying episodes this week."

"Any thoughts, images come to you while you were in this state?" I asked.

"I didn't pay much attention to that. It didn't seem relevant."

"My thought is that data exist that might be helpful in understanding what has been bothering you. It might lie in dreams or even the thoughts or images that come up in the relaxed state. Maybe we could do that here in session to see if there is anything that comes into your consciousness," I said, ready to go "data mining."

"To be honest, I am not sure I want to get at anything more. I feel better, and maybe it is better not to open Pandora's box right now." I understood his reluctance, but I also knew that there was something he was deeply sad about and that it would return at some point. I wondered if I should wait to pursue this. Maybe I should let him have his recovery, feel some control, and then when the deep sadness eventually came back, maybe he would return. This was always the dilemma about how and when to work with the resistance. Do you confront it, or let it be?

"Michael, can you talk to me about what might happen if we open Pandora's box?"

"Sorry, Fred. I can feel myself just not wanting to do it. I am afraid that we will end up back into the crying, and that feels dangerous to me. You helped me, and that is what I wanted. Thank you."

I felt stymied. I knew there was more, but he was saying this was as far as he wanted to take it. We had yet to talk about his marriage, which he had initially alluded to as being pretty dull and moribund.

"Okay. The relaxation tool seems to be working for you. I do want you to know that if something does come up, do not hesitate to contact me. I mean that." This was my way of saying that if the Band-Aid doesn't work, I am ready to go deeper.

"I hope I don't have to. Thanks for everything."

So I let him walk out the door, knowing that it was unlikely I'd see him again. Something was definitely causing his emotional outbursts, but he did not seem ready or willing to go any further in his exploration.

In the following weeks, I periodically thought about Michael and wondered how he managed to deal with all the problems that a dean must face, including budget and, most important, people. When I was a dean I found that the people problems were the most vexing, so I wondered if some of what triggered Michael might be some of the personal and professional issues students, faculty, and other administrators might bring to the table.

It was the middle of June, around 6 months after our initial sessions, that Michael contacted me. I was getting ready to head up to the World Series of Poker in Las Vegas on my annual quest to play the best in the world. It was my fantasy that I would someday earn a bracelet, the gold standard of excellence in poker. In my daydream I imagined myself taking down the Senior 50 Years and Over crown. Michael had left me a message that he needed to see me as soon as possible. I called him back and let him know I would be heading out of town for a week starting tomorrow. He asked if I could see him tonight. I relented and scheduled him for my last possible slot at 8 p.m.

## Overwhelmed by Losses

Michael was in a T-shirt and jeans. He had several days of stubble. His hair was not combed. He had a manic look and was more edgy in his movements than in our previous encounters.

"Fred, I needed to talk to you. It happened again."

"What happened?" I asked.

"You said if something comes up to call you. I know it has been a while. . . ." He paused. "Everything I have feared would happen is coming true."

"What do you mean?" He was talking as if I could read his mind, but I didn't know what he meant.

"Mom died yesterday. I didn't think I'd have such a strong reaction, but I couldn't stop crying."

"I'm sorry to hear of her passing. Crying at your mother's death seems really appropriate, Michael. You lost someone important to you."

"That's not all. Rebecca, my wife, told me she wanted a divorce. That happened this morning. I can't believe she would tell me just when I was getting the news of my mother. Rebecca said she was tired of me being so distant. I was totally taken by surprise." He shook his head. "There is more. Yesterday I was told that my contract was not going to be renewed. They want to go in a different direction in the dean's office. The only positive is that they offered to bring me back into the physics department. I didn't even know they were not happy with my performance."

"That is a lot of loss all at once," I responded. I was feeling overwhelmed for Michael. Intellectually, he seemed so naive about all that had come down on him, yet his emotional self had been picking up on the signals and anticipating the danger.

"I'm lost," was all he could say.

"Say more," I encouraged.

"I never thought this would happen. I didn't want to look at the reality of my life when I talked with you months ago. You wanted to dig deeper, and I didn't want to go there. I thought if we didn't open the box, then nothing could get out. I guess the unconscious part of me knew I was about to lose everything. I didn't want to face that."

"Like if you didn't mention it, it wouldn't happen?"

"Yes. I've done that my whole life with things that were outside of my control. I just shut them out and focused on the tasks I had to do. It worked most of the time, so I didn't question it."

"You feeling ready now to deal with your life?" I asked.

"What's left of it. . . . I am so alone now." Michael sobbed. I handed him the box of tissues. He kept repeating, "I am so alone."

"You have always been alone. You are just acutely aware of it now."

"You're right. I thought I could live in my own intellectual bubble. I never thought about the consequences. As a scientist, I should have known there would be some kind of reaction. I guess my depression has been trying to talk to me about what was happening. I didn't listen," he said in between sniffles.

"It is hard to buy that psychological equation when you haven't really had to pay attention to it," I replied.

"The message has been there my whole life. I just kept finding ways to drown it out until the dike broke. The message is clear now."

"The life you have described to me does sound lonely. Your childhood seemed lonely too," I added.

"I have nothing more to lose. I need to figure how I can move on from here. I don't want to go back to my old 'head in the sand' approach. I'm willing to start from scratch and rebuild."

"You have already started by being here today and being open emotionally. Let's keep it going. I have a spot for you in my schedule next week."

"What about the crying spells?"

"Michael, it is okay to cry. Use the exercises to relax if you need to, but grief needs to be released or it will build up even more."

"Like a boiling water that has no outlet."

"Exactly."

"I will survive."

"Yes. You will."

## Personal Reflection

- How does Michael's initial presentation impact you? What is your countertransference reaction to his highly intellectual vocabulary? How might you best connect with an individual who seems very disconnected from his emotions?
- What are your thoughts about helping a client with symptom relief when you know there are deeper issues contributing to his discomfort? How might you approach his fears about digging into his inner emotional life?
- Why do you think Michael's psychological defenses failed him when he was faced with multiple losses? Even though early therapy was focused on symptom relief, what was your reaction to him reaching out when he was overwhelmed? What are the implications of working with clients who seem reluctant to go deeper?

## What Makes Michael a Good Candidate for Group?

Michael has been insulated from deep emotional connection most of his life. The losses of his mother, wife, and job have opened the portal to his emotional depth. The uncontrolled crying was the manifestation of feeling loss, aloneness, and disconnection. Michael kept his distance from others through his intellect and focus on rationality. As someone who had experienced aloneness most of his life, he appears to have become used to emotional distance in his relationships. His need for connection had remained mostly unconscious until the losses in his life converged on him in a short time span.

Michael could use some emotional support, and a group of men can provide this for him. An emotionally intense group might overwhelm him, so he might need time to find a comfortable space in the group to share. Michael also needs practice with his interpersonal skills. By getting feedback from the group, he can enhance his ability to connect with others and increase his self-awareness. He is very attentive and will benefit from observing others sharing their experiences. Michael brings an intellectual orientation to the group that many of the men will know as ways they too distance themselves from their emotions to some degree. Michael will likely find some commonality with the men around the difficulty with emotions, as well as the common link of loss as a portal to depth.

# III

# DOING GROUP THERAPY WITH MEN

## INTRODUCTION: DOING GROUP THERAPY WITH MEN

> In my first year of the group I think what I appreciated most was the relief of not being all alone with my problems. Realizing that a good portion of my internal turmoil were "men's issues" opened new ways to react to myself and helped me re-sort myself out in my own mind. I think I also learned to appreciate the pain and bravery of others in the group.
>
> —A member of the men's group

It was 1981. The initial men's group I co-led was an experiment. I was struggling to stay in my first marriage, while pursuing my PhD in counseling at the University of Missouri. The world had flipped upside down in terms of male–female relationships from male "dominant" to female "in charge," and then to male "confused." Unlike my father's generation, I was far from being in charge in my primary relationship. Other guys were feeling it too. The culture of relationships had shifted to a power-sharing egalitarian model that most of us had not learned growing up.

Under the general heading of "What does it mean to be a man in this new era?" I imagined a "support" group for men who were in relationships with the empowered, assertive women of the early 1980s. With my best friend in graduate school, Sam Cochran, we got the go-ahead to create a group for men. We ran the weekly group out of the University Counseling Center. We had no idea where it would go or if it was even going to be helpful. Fortunately, the guys who were willing to join were pioneers themselves. They were going up against the norms of masculinity that said, "Keep your problems to yourself," "Figure things out on your own," and "Don't ask for help." But my hunch was on target. Much of what we discussed was about the changing rules of relationships and how we were supposed to see ourselves as men. I was a leader but also a participant. I began to look forward to the group sessions because every issue we addressed was one I needed to grapple with as much as anyone. How do you deal with your anger? Why do I define myself so much by my work? Is competition good or bad? Why is it so hard to share what is inside me? Will expressing all of my feelings make me weak? What does it mean to live a meaningful life as a man?

Over the many ensuing years of being a men's group participant and facilitator, I gained a sense of how being a part of a group like this was beneficial. One of the central core principles about why a men's group worked was that it brought together isolated individuals. While men seem to be trained by our culture to tough it out alone, the group asked them to share who they were with each other. Men got to be both the recipients of and givers of emotional support. They told stories and heard about the adventures of each other's life journeys. They found the common themes to discuss and relate to, and in the process felt less alone, and more connected to the universal experience of being a man.

The group also served as a communications laboratory. I had observed that often men relied on women to facilitate their emotional expression. In the group there were no women to rely on for their interpersonal expertise. The group encouraged men to speak and share in a language that was right for them. Often this meant more storytelling, speaking in metaphors, and even confronting each other when disagreements arose. My role as facilitator was often to encourage, model, and break down interpersonal conflicts so they could be worked out. Many men had learned to avoid conflict or try to win intellectual arguments, rather than figuring out what the conflict might be about from a psychological perspective. The group helped to provide context and a variety of voices to any given dilemma.

Over the years, the men's group I have led in Redlands, California, has changed composition dozens of times. Some men worked on themselves in the group for a year, while others have been a part of it for more than 20 years. The mix of new and old members added a club-like feel to our encounters. It was clear that doing some individual work prior to entry was helpful in utilizing the benefits of the group experience. Each man brought a unique perspective. If you had run into any of our members out on the street, you wouldn't peg them as being candidates for individual or group therapy. They represented "everyman" in terms of being tough and strong on the outside but rich, deep, and diverse on the inside. Unlike the stereotypes in the media, men have a depth of experience that is hidden beneath the surface personality. Like fashion, they look, dress, and act the part of masculinity as it is defined by culture. Most observe these outer expressions of manhood and know that their own conformity is a fake. It is as if they are actors in the public space, defining themselves by the superficial markings of what it means to be a man. Ironically, each man feels alone with his inner thoughts and conflicts: "Surely, no one else feels like I do." That is one of the surprise insights that the men's group has provided.

The issues revealed in individual therapy find new outlets in the group. Rather than just hear the therapeutic words of a helping professional, the men supported by a "Greek chorus" of fellow travelers. Through group interaction, they face dilemmas and opportunities to grow as individuals, but they also feel a more a universal connection to each other and humanity. The issues that make up the core of group learning include

- *What does it mean to be a man?* The group inevitably engages in an ongoing critique about the damaging aspects of the masculine role, as well as acknowledging what is positive about being a man.
- *Public self and private self.* The group encourages men to reflect on how they differ in expectation and behavior when they are in public settings versus more private and intimate environments. The intimacy of a men's group lets men be real with what they are feeling, whether it be anger, sadness, or laughter.
- *Identity.* The group allows men to define themselves to other men but also explore the projections and stereotypes around race, sexuality, gender, and culture. The consequent understanding of not only how one is perceived but also how he thinks about himself in this realm is revealing for the individual and the group cohesion.
- *Mind–body connection.* Health issues, self-care, mortality, and the psychological and physical consequences of living a life of stress make their way into the group discussions.
- *Self-judgment, shame, and self-compassion.* A common theme for most men is the harsh internal criticism for not living up to ideal masculine scripts and the perceived expectations of others in their environment. Many of these messages come from traumatic childhood experiences and incidences of betrayal and loss of innocence in growing up. Many times the relationship with one's father stirs much of the internal dialogue. The healing in the group often occurs through internalizing the compassion the members show each other.
- *Loss.* The men in the group have a chance to revisit past losses, including relationships and lost opportunities that have been minimized and forgotten.
- *Interpersonal skills.* Through facilitated interaction men learn to "own" their projections onto others, and in the process realize that the other men can provide them with anchors about themselves. Listening, supporting, and learning to confront in a caring way translate to outside relationship enhancement.

- *Meaning in life.* At the core of many group sessions is a theme of finding or rediscovering one's purpose. In the group, men get to reflect on their lives, rekindle passion, and remind themselves of what is most important.
- *Finding the fire inside.* The group collective supports freeing up one's ability to act, to take risks, to face difficult emotions, to laugh, and to change life situations that keep one shut down. The validation a man receives from his men's group companions for taking steps to be the man he wants to be is priceless.

You have already met in the preceding chapters the mosaic of men (whose identities have been changed to preserve confidentiality) who met for group every Wednesday night for 9 months, and included a camping weekend together. The upcoming chapters highlight how Deepening psychotherapy can be applied to the group modality with men and will give you an up-close observation of the group process and how various issues are manifested and facilitated.

# 10

# Building Trust

## *Scenes From the Early Stages of the Men's Group*

In this chapter and in Chapters 11 and 12, I describe a men's group at different stages of the Deepening process. Three new members joined my group in the fall of 2016, so to accommodate them, the group had to spend some time on interactions that primarily built trust. Topics of our October and November conversations described here included basics such as boundaries and expectations for group start and end times and how "permeable" the walls of the therapy room would be. Would the men extend their friendship outside of therapy, and if so, what would they agree was okay to talk about without therapist facilitation? Veteran members of the group modeled how to be vulnerable to others in, for example, a Gestalt empty-chair dialogue in front of the group. They also modeled their trust in other members by disclosing personal information and by introducing topics that stirred up strong opinions and emotions.

### BREAKING THE SURFACE

Kean, Michael, and Tony joined the group in October 2016. The other seven had been part of the men's group from 1 to 10 years.

"Where is everyone? I thought the group started at 7 p.m.," announced Kean to the two other new members, who made it into the room on time. Kean looked at me as if I was to blame. Of course, I could have been a

http://dx.doi.org/10.1037/0000132-011
*Deepening Group Psychotherapy With Men: Stories and Insights for the Journey*,
by F. E. Rabinowitz

no-nonsense leader and made some kind of authoritarian rule about not letting anyone in after 7. But this was Southern California, land of freeways and traffic jams, especially during rush hour. The men were coming from as far away as Santa Monica, Palm Springs, and Lake Arrowhead. It wasn't so easy to get here on time. The best I could do is start at 7 p.m. and let those who got here early begin. But it was true: The new guys made it on time, whereas those who had been to the group in previous years did not, and that should probably be brought up if it continued to be an issue.

I started chatting with the three new members about how their weeks had been. All of them knew me from individual therapy, so I was the glue that held them together at this point. The other men already in the room were Michael and Tony. Michael did not give away much in his face. Because group for this year had started only 3 weeks earlier, he was still feeling it out. He looked uncomfortable, but no more than usual. Tony was a new member too. He was a bit more laid-back. I focused first on Kean, who could be prickly. Kean and I had met regularly for 3 years before he started the group.

"What's going on for you, Kean?" I asked.

"Just a little frustrated that these guys aren't more committed to being on time."

"Why don't you say something to them?" interjected Tony, his big tattooed arms crossed in front of him.

"I probably should, but I don't know them that well," replied Kean.

"It certainly seems to be bothering you," I added. We were interrupted by the sound of a door opening, some loud voices, and laughter. Four group members arrived together. Tony smiled. "Here they come. The four Musketeers." Kean got quiet.

Into the room walked Peter, Justin, Carlton, and Ray. It was good for me to hear Peter laughing. Peter had been battling depression and isolation. Justin, wearing a Dodgers cap, found a seat in the corner of the room. Carlton started stacking pillows to create a throne for his massive body in one of the room corners. We all sit on the floor with an array of pillows giving us some comfort. Being on the ground is grounding. No one is sitting higher than anyone else. Ray, wearing his long gray hair down, made eye contact with the three guys and me and smiled as he found a seat next to Kean.

"Hey, everybody. Sorry we were late. The waitress wasn't accommodating to our need to get out of there." The four guys had been at a local tavern, having a bite to eat and catching up before the group officially began.

Although some group therapists would discourage this kind of pregroup meeting, I have observed its benefits. The downside is that by creating a "pregame" subgroup, there is the potential for them to defend one another and withhold information. I addressed this by asking the guys to make sure they brought into the group anything they spoke about that was relevant to themselves or the group. So far, they had been good about raising issues that were discussed at dinner. I also liked it because it was another way for men to feel camaraderie. But I didn't like that not everyone was able to go, so it felt a bit exclusive, but all had been explicitly invited.

Two members were coming from far away and often showed up late. Lee was coming in from Orange County, and Neil often had patients in his medical practice right up to 7 p.m. Kevin had called in earlier that he was not going to make it tonight.

Early in the process of a new group, I use structured exercises to help the guys move to a deeper level. Later there is enough material generated by members sharing openly, as well as by our evolving group dynamics. Tonight I had brought in a starter that asked them to confront a bit of their discomfort with one another, given the new members' short time together.

"I want each of you to look around and choose a person in the group with whom you are a bit uncomfortable or don't know well. Once you pick, reveal something about yourself that you would like that man to know about you. Then you can ask a question of them. Make sense?"

No one moved or talked. The silence hung in the air. One of the veteran group members looked at me. Maybe they didn't understand. I didn't exactly plead, but I did project with my eyes some desire for a response. Just as Peter was ready to speak, Kean cleared his throat. Peter stopped.

"I have been depressed most of my life. It sucks. I work every day to try to be okay with myself. I wonder if I'm really capable of love," Kean admitted to the group and added, "I do feel a bit uncomfortable around the guys who came in late. Can I ask what you guys were talking about before the group?"

"Why don't you ask one of the guys specifically?" I directed.

"Okay. Peter, what do you get out of meeting before the group with the other guys?"

"You don't know me that well, Kean, but I have been super isolated. I just like being around people. I like the guys who come out. You'd be welcome to enjoy a meal before the group with us."

"Why were you so isolated?" asked Kean in a very direct manner. Peter hesitated. The guys who knew him anticipated his revelation by averting their eyes. Peter cleared his throat and fumbled with his phone before he spoke.

"My daughter and wife were killed in a car accident a couple of years ago," he said in a monotone voice.

"Oh, my God," mouthed Kean. "I am so sorry. I don't know what to say."

"There isn't much to say. I'm not sure God has much to do with it." The traffic noise from the street was the only sound in the room. Kean's face softened. "I'm glad you said something, Peter. I didn't mean to pry. It helps me get where you are coming from more."

"We'd love to have you come with us for dinner before group. That goes for everyone here," Peter announced as a small smile formed, overshadowing the heaviness of his disclosure. I liked that he was making the predinner invitation explicit. It also showed me that Peter was feeling more acceptance of the tragedy, even though its power would be with him for the rest of his life. "Can I ask you something, Kean?" queried Peter.

"Sure."

"Why aren't you happy? Seems like you have your family intact. What is it that makes you so dissatisfied with your life, Kean?"

"Compared with your experience, I should be happy. But I have had some tragedy in my life too. It's not so fresh, but I think it set the tone."

"What do you mean?" asked Peter.

"My parents split when I was a kid. I was pretty neglected. I never saw much of my dad. He pretty much checked out."

"Sorry to hear that. My dad fortunately has been around for me throughout this whole ordeal. I owe him a lot. I'm sure there is a story there about your dad," he added.

Kean seemed unprepared to go deep, especially given his dad's death by suicide. "I am not sure I can talk about it right now." His question was based on some irritation about the pregroup dinner had led to an openness he wasn't quite expecting. This is not uncommon in a group that has both new and veteran members. Those who have been in group often socialize and model what can be shared in this setting.

"That's okay. I appreciate what you have shared. You're welcome any time to go hang with the guys. I hope you know that," continued Peter.

"Thanks."

"Fathers is a tough subject," shared Carlton. "My dad died when I was young. I don't remember much of him, sadly. I think my life would have been different had he been around."

"How old were you when he died?" asked Kean.

"About 10. How about you?"

"Me too. I was pretty young when he left, and then I heard later that he died." Kean couldn't bring himself to admit to the group that his dad's death was a suicide.

"You two aren't the only ones who didn't really know your dads. My dad was never there. I met him a few times, but I grew up totally without a dad," said Justin.

"My dad died a few years ago," shared Michael, who seemed to perk up in the discussion about lost fathers.

"My dad is alive but on dialysis. He has lost so much of his health, but I still talk to him," said Tony.

"What about you, Ray?" asked Tony.

"My dad and I never really got along. He was pretty authoritarian. Not my style. He is still around, but I haven't seen him in a while. Last time we talked, he didn't listen to me. He just continued to turn me off," Ray responded with disdain.

"Fathers is a pretty big topic," I interjected. "What do you imagine your dad would say to you about being in this men's group?"

"Ha. My dad would probably say, 'Why do you need that?'" replied Ray.

"What would be your answer, Ray?" asked Tony.

"I guess I would want to tell him that it is good to get support. That the lone wolf approach to being a man doesn't work for me."

"I like that answer," said Tony. "My dad is a heavy-duty Catholic. He would say, 'All we need is God.' I have done the 'go at it alone' so long that it almost killed me. Thanks to working with Fred, I realize I can't pull myself up alone. I love this group for that reason."

The group was staying on the surface. We were early in the year, but many of the veteran group members were open to going deeper. The new guys needed to make the leap without freaking themselves out. My dad had died 10 years ago, but not before letting me in on every question I had about his life. I felt fortunate to get some closure, but I still miss his presence in my life. Kean, Michael, and Tony were the members who needed to break the ice. In individual therapy, all three had made a lot of progress, but in the group, even more trust was needed before they were going to bare their souls.

Justin stepped up. "I feel the most uncomfortable with you, Michael. I'll say something, and maybe it will let you and I connect better. While we are talking about dads, I thought I'd share that I actually have the potential to have a relationship with my dad, and I haven't taken it. My dad has tried to contact me. He gave me financial support when I was younger, but I was so pissed that he wasn't there at crucial points in my life that I have blown him off."

Michael looked at me to get permission to speak. I nodded to him.

"Justin. I wish my dad were still alive. He died a few years ago. He was very introverted and quiet. I think I am a lot like him."

"Michael, why don't you first let Justin know you heard what he said," I interrupted, trying to encourage Michael's practice upgrading his communication skills to make better interpersonal connections.

"Oh, sorry. Justin, I hear you say that you have mixed feelings about getting to know your dad. I know I am not you. But I would jump on the chance to get to know him. You never know what you might learn from him."

"I second that," said Carlton. "I was too young to remember much, but as a Black man in this world, I wish I had a father figure who understood that reality. It is not easy to navigate it out there."

Lee walked through the door just as Carlton was sharing. "I'm sorry I'm late. I am missing some good stuff. I have no idea what the context is, but Carlton, I can feel for you, man. All these good White guys can't quite get what it's like to be Black in America these days."

"Dude. Thanks for the support. We are talking about fathers," replied Carlton. Lee smiled a bit sheepishly and sat slowly on some pillows as Michael replied to Justin.

"My dad was an academic like me. He was the smartest person I know. It's not like we talked a lot, but we definitely thought alike. Very rational. . . . Very scientific."

"I can tell you miss him," said Justin.

"For sure," replied Michael. "Not sure he helped me very much with my people skills, though. My ex seemed to tolerate me for a while until she couldn't hang with my nonemotional style. My parents seemed to be okay with that style. My mom was also a professor, so it worked. I realize now that I can't just see the world through my rational lens only. I am missing a lot."

"I know you said you were rational, but do you have feelings of sadness about not being able to ever talk to your dad anymore?" asked Justin.

"I am working on feeling more, rather than letting it all build up. For a while I couldn't stop crying. Right now, I think I am still holding back some because I don't know everyone so well in here," Michael replied.

"Well, I hope you get there in terms of trust. Some of the best stuff that happens in this group comes about when we can be real with each other. But I hold back too. This father thing is big for me. I'm still not quite ready to move towards him, but some part of me knows it's the right thing to do," replied Justin.

"My father is a prick. I can't share with him anything about my life," injected Ray, unable to contain his feelings anymore during the conversation.

"That's pretty strong, Ray. You want to say more?" I asked.

"This dad shit is really stirring me up. When I got diagnosed with cancer, I tried to tell my dad what was happening. You know what he said? He told me that I probably brought it on myself. This guy is a doctor, for heaven's sake." Ray had a lot of energy that was begging for release.

"Ray. You up for the punching bag? You seem ready for it," I said, pointing to the bag hanging in the corner of the room. Ray had done this before. He put on the yellow boxing gloves. Carlton stood behind the bag holding it, to keep it from swinging too much. Ray began pounding with his fists.

"Hit it harder, Ray," encouraged Carlton, whose face was in his sight. Ray sped up his swings.

"Put some words on it," I encouraged. His grunts began to get louder.

"Cold bastard. Fuck you," he yelled and repeated. The members of the group encouraged him. "Get 'em, Ray." "Kick his ass." "Keep it going, Ray."

I looked around and saw that only Michael was pulled back, the emotion too intense. As Ray started to slow down after a few minutes, the anger on his face turned to tears.

"What is it, Ray? What's so sad?" asked Peter. Ray slumped, supported by both Peter and Justin, their arms cradling him like the trainers in his corner between rounds in a prizefight.

"I needed him. I rejected him, but couldn't he see how much pain I was in? I could have used a real father. I am sorry for being a fucked-up son, but you didn't have to abandon me when I needed you." Soon Ray was talking as if his father were in the room with us. "Dad, why did you keep your distance from me?"

"Ray, what would he say if he was here? Be your dad for a minute," I directed him, using the Gestalt empty-chair technique.

"Ray. You rejected me first. What did I do to hurt you, son?" Ray said.

"Ray. Respond to him as you."

"Dad, you were always so much in your own world. You were the important doctor who had no time for me. What were you afraid of? Was I that much of a pain in the ass?"

"Ray, what do you think he was afraid of?" I asked. Ray hesitated. He sagged into the two men behind him.

With an otherworldly strength and wisdom, he stated, "My dad was afraid of closeness. I was too emotional for him. I demanded his full engagement and he couldn't give it to me. That was his loss . . . and mine."

"Anything else get stirred up?" I asked.

"I feel some guilt. I heard Justin talk about his dad just sending money and not being around. I hate to admit it, but I am that father too. You guys don't know this, but I did not see my daughter the first 10 years of her life. I just reconnected with her recently when this cancer thing happened. I'm not so sure I have a right to be so indignant when I did the same thing to my daughter."

"I'm glad to hear you say that, Ray. I wonder if my dad feels like that with me," said Justin.

"We have to stop here," I interrupted. "We have more meetings to get to work on some of these issues."

Arms on one another's shoulders, the guys made a circle around Ray. They closed in for a squeeze of support. Ray, eyes shut, let himself be held up by the group. After a couple of minutes, he opened his blue eyes and smiled. Spontaneously, each of the guys reflected back to him their own smiles and eye contact.

## Commentary

These interactions in an early group session were significant for several reasons. New group members had the opportunity to share, and the veteran members could begin some psychological work. The discomfort embodied by Kean soon was transformed to empathy when Peter revealed his reason for being in the group. Although Kean wasn't ready for this type of revelation, it did change the group dynamics. Kean's projection about the veteran members "not caring" became an opening for these experienced members to display some of the work that could be done in this setting. As the discussion moved to feelings about fathers, dads became a universal topic that allowed for a gamut of reactions. This discussion also brought all of the new members into the conversation. Although not everyone was willing to go deep making sense of their father relationships, Ray's readiness to work out some of his anger physically modeled some of what could happen in the group. Underneath his anger was hurt at not being seen. This discussion also stirred up some deep feeling in Justin, who realized that Ray could be feeling what his father felt toward him. The group hug gave Ray some of the support he needed and allowed the men an opportunity to experience unexpected closeness around a difficult topic.

## Practical Tips

- Our group meets for 2 hours on 1 night a week for 9 months. Although not everyone can make every group, the process depends upon continuity week to week. Many of the issues and themes will recycle themselves and build upon previous work.

- An ideal group size is eight to 12 members. This allows individuals to participate, observe, and reflect on the ongoing interactions.
- Some groups start fresh with new members, but I have found that a mix of new and old members allows for some socialization to how the group works in terms of how to get one's voice into the conversation. The mixed group also models communication skills and how to share more vulnerable disclosures.
- The circular seating arrangement on the floor allows for everyone to be seen and signifies that the group discussion is egalitarian and nonhierarchical. Because the members do not sit in regular chairs, the group space is less formal than in a common work environment.
- Although the subgrouping of those who go to dinner before group can be problematic, there is a counterargument for its presence. These members actively invite others to come with them, so it is not exclusive. They also are conscientious about bringing relevant disclosures into the group. Most members would like to be a part of the pregroup social time, but it is not required or encouraged by me, because some may be unable to afford meals out or may not have the time to engage.
- Because members come into the group with some individual therapy experience, many have been exposed to some of the techniques and exercises, such as the one used with Ray. Others need to be explicitly told in pregroup interviews about the nature of potential interventions in the group. I usually explain what the intervention will be in the moment and get permission from the individual before enacting it.

## TALKING ABOUT RACE AND POLITICS

When the group met in November 2016, talk turned immediately to the recent election results and what effects the country's new leadership (the Donald Trump administration) might have.

"I can't believe it. What has happened to our damn country?" exclaimed Lee, with more passion that I had seen in him during his time in the group. "I thought after all these years with Obama, we were making some progress. I'm in shock."

"Amen, brother," added Carlton. "This is a backlash. I kind of expected it."

"If it is impacting you, we should probably talk about the meaning of this for each of us," I interjected. "Unspoken resentment won't be good for our communication. That would suck."

"Well, I can't imagine who would have wanted the guy in here," added Neil. "But I don't want us to be divided as a group. Is there anyone who wants to argue for why the billionaire is good?"

"I do," said Tony, after a brief pause. "I own my own business. Trump is a business guy, and I think it was important to make it less hard for us entrepreneurs and small businessmen. Having said that, I could also see him needing the men's group for some self-reflection." Tony tried to make a joke, but it went flat in the group.

"Tony, he said a lot of shit about Hispanics and Mexicans. Didn't that bother you as someone who is of Mexican descent?" asked Kean, who seemed ready to engage tonight.

"I heard it. There are some bad people out there who came across the border illegally. That's who needs to go," replied Tony, his large forearms folded across his chest in defense position.

"But that's such a stereotype. How would anyone know if you were legal or illegal if you have the Hispanic look? Aren't you concerned for you or your kids?" scolded Kean, with an air of self-righteousness.

"Of course. But I will kick anyone's ass who messes with me that way. I've taught my kids that too. I know the guy is far from perfect, but we could loosen up the strings a bit on how much interference the government inflicts on our lives."

"Whoa. I'm more pissed about the racial stuff. I'm not sure that you guys actually know what it is like to be Black, even in California," Lee retorted. "How many times have you been stopped in the neighborhood?" He looked around. The room silenced. "Anyone?"

Kevin, a police officer, shifted uncomfortably and looked as if he might want to say something in response to Lee's question. He remained quiet.

Carlton smiled and raised his hand. "Four times this year, but there is still a month to go," he joked.

"Let's see, between the brother and I, we have been stopped 10 times this year. Lifetime, maybe 25 for me. . . . How about you, Carlton?"

"Sounds about right, Lee. I'm not as old as you."

"Wow. I had no idea," shared Michael. "I have some Chinese heritage, but I have never had any of those routine traffic stops."

"Me either," said Peter.

"I've had a few from my dope-smoking days," replied Ray. "I sometimes get the long hair stare from cops, even now."

"Lee, talk about what this stirs up for you," I said.

"It pisses me off. I have bent over backwards to make sure White people feel comfortable around me. I am not one of those angry, glaring Black men who try to scare you. I have been working in mainly White settings. Now I'm wondering. I am not sure I trust that they understand me as much as I gave them credit," said Lee with conviction.

"What about in here, Lee? Are you saying that we might not fully understand?" I asked. I redirected the conversation to our group, worried that there could be a simmering rift if this didn't get some airtime.

"Well, I like everyone here. I don't think my group brothers are the problem."

I looked at Kevin and nodded, encouraging him to share given what I knew about his profession. Kevin looked directly at Lee. "You know I care a lot about you, Lee. I hate that you have been racially profiled. That is not right. I can't defend some of my fellow officers. Some are just assholes. I can say that most are not. I know that doesn't help you feel any less harassed."

"Appreciate your honesty, Kevin. I've gotten to know you, and I know you have integrity," said Lee.

"What about Tony? He was the one who stirred you up," injected Kean.

"Lee, I can take the feedback. I do want to hear about your anger," said Tony, holding out an olive branch.

"This is not easy. I am so used to getting along with everyone. Something about this blatant narcissist being our president rubs me the wrong way. I've encountered my share of racists, but he seems clueless. It feels personal to me, Tony, that you would support someone like this." Tony maintained eye contact, but his arms remained folded across his chest.

"I don't know, Lee. The guy just says it like it is. No bullshit. It's not filtered through the lens of political correctness. I'm not saying you are some politically correct guy or anything," Tony replied.

"What are you saying, Tony?" Lee's breathing deepened. The muscles tensed on his forearms. I noticed that Kevin, who had that cop awareness for violence, began to inch toward Tony and Lee.

"Look, Lee. It's not personal. I like you. It has nothing to do with you. I just wanted to change things up. He's a jackass. I'm not denying that, but he represents some different ways of thinking."

"I can respect that, but this is deeply personal to me. My grandfather was beat during the Jim Crow era in Mississippi. My mother told me about how scared she was growing up there. This feels like regression. I felt proud that we had progressed to a place where everyone had a shot at being successful. Now I face a guy who woke up on third base and thinks he hit a triple. Even if he is aware of his big, fat, rich White privilege, he doesn't care. He thinks he deserves it. Barack had to be perfect as a Black man—nonthreatening but smart and fair."

"I hadn't thought so deeply about it, but I really get what the brother is saying," interrupted Carlton. "I have also been one of those guys who has had to live in two worlds with a White mother and Black father. The president was on my level, even though personally I have not lived up to my potential. He has. I respect that."

"Lee, the pain you express around your grandfather and just how much it takes for you to have to be aware of the color of your skin seems exhausting," I interjected.

Lee relaxed his fist. "I know it is not about you, Tony. This shit has been piled up for a while. I have pushed down so many comments and stares in my lifetime. When I was in the sports industry, there was some sensitivity, but there was a lot of outright racism that I laughed off."

"Still hurt underneath," I said.

"Yes. I don't like to show this side of myself. Most people don't get to see what's under my tough, Black exterior."

"How does it feel to do that here?" I continued.

"I feel a bit of relief, but my damn back is starting to act up. You and I have talked about this. It is usually when I get stressed. I tense up, and my body just locks down. I want to relax it. Looks like I might be over the edge."

Lee and I had worked hard on awareness of his body and how stress makes it worse. We had also talked about how to prepare for stressful situations so that he was ready for them. He seemed to be ready for this one.

"You know, Lee, I do the same thing around White people. I go out of my way to make them feel comfortable with me. It does take a lot of energy to be the righteous man of color," said Tony, who seemed to be looking for common ground. Tony was sensitive to Lee's pain. He didn't want the conflict. Lee, who had his hand on his back, looked up at Tony. "Man, I don't want to fight with you. I needed you and everyone else to know, I'm not cool with this rich, narcissistic dude as the leader of the Western world. Normally, I would have kept it to myself and steamed. You know I get depressed really easy." Lee looked at me and continued. "I've been working to be more expressive. The alternative is not good for me."

"I totally relate to that, Lee," said Tony. "I also struggle with depression and anxiety. It sucks."

"I wonder if the whole Trump thing is just a way for people to express their anger and frustration. He provided a target," opined Michael.

"He certainly has pissed off people too. It's like a collective 'fuck you' on both sides," said Ray, who seemed engrossed in the conflict.

"We could get into an analysis of the whole phenomenon, but I think it is important to take meaning from our emotional reactions here. Usually things we focus on in the outside reality are triggers for past traumatic events. I wonder if our group dynamic mirrors some of the disconnect that was in the election," I added.

"On a personal level, I think Lee and Carlton reminded me of my privilege as a middle-class White man," replied Kean.

"In what way?" I asked.

"As much as I want to identify with everyone, I haven't been stopped driving my car because of what I look like. I mostly am oblivious to the crap that people take and just worry about myself. Lee, Carlton, I am sorry for not being more aware of the bullshit out there. Wake-up call for me," Kean added.

"I know you can't really know what it's like out there for us brothers and anyone else who doesn't fit the mold, but I do appreciate your support. Thanks, man," Lee responded.

Several of the members nodded in response to Lee's words.

"Let's keep it real in here. That's what I like about this group," Ray added, speaking as if he had a voice for the collective.

## Commentary

This group brought conflict to the forefront for the members. I, too, was triggered by the election of a man who seemed to represent a backward notion of masculinity. Parsing my reactions as a person, and separately as a leader, required taking a step back to understand what this had stirred up in me. For me as a man, the election reinforced a stereotyped notion of who I should be from the traditional perspective outlined decades ago by David and Brannon (1976): "the big wheel," "the sturdy oak," "give 'em hell," and "no sissy stuff." I have spent my professional career challenging these suppositions. As a leader, I had an obligation to understand deeply each one of my clients' perspectives, including those with whom I might personally disagree. In this session it was as important to get where Tony was coming from, as it was to empathize with Lee's perspective as an African American man who has done battle with racism. My role as a leader meant that we needed to talk about the issues, personalize them, and deal with what they meant in terms of our dynamics in the group setting.

The election results led us to discuss the racial, ethnic, and cultural differences in the group. Although the topic might have been stirred up at a later time, this discussion was important in laying out these issues as the group worked on a more nuanced and in-depth understanding of one another. It seemed important for Tony and Lee to dialog respectfully and acknowledge their differences but not make it an all-or-nothing proposition. Kean's supportive words seemed to work toward inclusion, when the group potentially could have gone off the rails in divisiveness.

## Practical Tips

- Anticipating how cultural and political events will impact the content of a given group is often impossible. If a member brings in a reaction to an outside situation, it is important to see if it has relevance to the dynamics within the group. The November 2016 presidential election clearly was a lightning rod to discuss race and privilege.

- Even though I may have had a different agenda for the night's work, the emotional energy brought in around the election made it poignant. This was an opportunity for Lee to share and not hold back his emotions, a goal he had for himself in the group. The topic also exposed division within the group, even among the men of color.

- Race is always hard to discuss, and White privilege is an even more difficult topic. Often, men want to deny their own racism or rationalize that they do not feel "that way" toward individuals they know who are of a different race. The group leader needs to be fair and empathic but also clear about where he or she stands on these issues to best facilitate. The intersection of masculinity with race, socioeconomic status, and often sexual orientation is important to address, but it is not always clear when it should be front and center.

- In this situation, the election provided an opening for the expression of opinion but also exposure of each man's schema around race. This kind of discussion could have happened later in the group process, when newer members were more integrated and trusting. However, it does have the impact of exposing a conflict that pushes the group to face its tendency to avoid topics that might jeopardize the sense of belonging inclusiveness among its members. This can be the kind of discussion that takes the group to a deeper level.

# 11

# Deepening the Connections

## *Scenes From the Middle Stage of the Men's Group*

In the middle stage, men's groups can explore weighty topics such as shame, loss, resentment, and desire. They can also withstand a higher level of interpersonal conflict. By this point they have been together long enough to have at least a taste of authenticity and its rewards. Group members in this stage may be more concerned with keeping one another accountable to their stated goals, or ensuring others' words are honest, than with being nice to each other. The vignettes described in this chapter illustrate what Deepening group psychotherapy might look like 3 to 4 months after integrating new members into the group.

### FINDING MOJO IN THE SHADOWS

Coming into the holiday season in December, I anticipated that some members of my group would feel an extra edge to their depression, or maybe an extra pressure to make huge, impossible-to-fulfill resolutions for the New Year. I wanted them to talk about where they find their "mojo," their energy and passion, even if traditional holiday merrymaking didn't feel like an option for them.

"What makes you feel most alive?" I asked the group. I was hoping to spark a discussion about energy and how we block ourselves from being "all in" more of the time. As I looked around the room, I got mixed signals. Some of

http://dx.doi.org/10.1037/0000132-012
*Deepening Group Psychotherapy With Men: Stories and Insights for the Journey,*
by F. E. Rabinowitz

the guys smiled. Others looked down, maybe trying to access the last time they felt their mojo. I encouraged each man to share his answer, whether it was something he was currently feeling or not. The idea of the prompt was to think about what brought passion into one's life and then what might be blocking it.

Justin started. He looked around the circle and laughed. "You guys know what I love and what makes me feel most alive and engaged, right?"

"Besides poker?" cried out Neil with a smile.

"I hadn't really thought of anything else," Justin replied.

"What else might there be, Justin?" I asked.

"Doc, I know you love poker too. I guess it would be finding a woman who could tolerate me. So far, I haven't had any takers," he joked.

"What stops you from finding that person?" asked Neil. The smile disappeared from Justin's face. "I'm not sure I am ready. I have my hands full taking care of my mom and trying to make a living. Maybe I don't make the time for it."

"I can relate to that statement," said Kevin. "In my imagination, I would love to be with a soul mate, but my motivation is pretty low. I see lots of attractive women, yet I tend to run the other way. I guess I still feel burned by my ex-wife. I just seem to shut down. I wish it wasn't that way."

"That sounds really painful," said Kean. "I know what it is like to shut down."

I thought about following up with Kean but also didn't want to turn the attention away from Kevin, who was being more open than I had seen in the past few sessions.

"Kevin, anything else make you feel alive?" I asked.

"You guys are going to laugh or get pissed off, I bet."

"Go ahead," I said encouragingly.

"I love my job being a cop. I love the challenge in being able to bust people who think they won't get caught. The other thing I love is reading. Leave me with a good novel, or historical nonfiction, and I will be totally engaged for a long time."

"Me too," said Michael. "I was trying to think about what got me going. I love science fiction and will read anything related to space or space travel. I'm like Kevin. I could spend the whole weekend reading a book. I probably shouldn't do that, but that's honest."

Michael had also been quiet. It seemed important to also keep him in the conversation.

"Anything else?" I asked.

"Playing the piano. I can get lost working on classical pieces. There is something transcendent about music for me." Several members of the group nodded. I hoped that this attention would reinforce Michael to share, not just now but on a more regular basis.

"I can picture you doing that," said Ray. "I love music too. I play some guitar, but I really dig listening to music. I love jam bands and finding new music. I could probably get lost doing that all day. In fact, I think I may do too much of that. But seriously, I agree in a major way with Justin and Kevin around the serious relationship issue. Man, I want it in fantasy but certainly don't follow through very well." The underlying theme of wishing for a soul mate seemed to pervade the more overt topic of what brings you energy. There was a definite approach—avoidance to the relationship theme. I was curious as to where this was taking us as a group. It is a significant topic.

"Well, guys, I wish I had some of your restraint. I think about women a lot and seem to be more motivated by chasing tail than anything else. I like my work, but the scent of a new woman in my life is intoxicating," said Neil, his eyes closed, the corner of his mouth upturned. This was not covert for Neil, who readily acknowledged his pursuit of women as a mojo booster.

"Get out of here, dude," said Justin, half-joking. "Man, I don't want to hear your stories. They make me envious."

"Listen, it is not hard to jump on a dating site and go out on a date. It might do you some good," Neil countered.

"Maybe, but I do have standards," Justin replied. Kevin turned his head away. Something about the lightness of Neil's comments about women seemed to shut him down. I knew I would have to address this dynamic between Kevin and Neil before it became corrosive. Before I could follow up, Lee took the floor.

"Well, I've been thinking about all this stuff you guys have been saying. I used to be so into sports, like football and basketball, that the question would have been a no-brainer. It almost causes me pain to think about how much I made those two sports my life. Now I wish I could find something that even came close. You know, since I stopped, I have not really been that amped about anything. I should be more into my beautiful wife, I guess, but . . ." Lee's voice trailed off. He had the full attention of the group.

"But what?" Peter asked.

Lee hesitated, then said, "Most of you guys know I struggle with depression and chronic pain, but it also impacts how I perform sexually. Making love to my wife would have been near the top of my most passionate moments. Lately, this hasn't been happening. Man, I have a lot of shame around this." Lee put his head in his hands and blocked out the group.

"I have that too, Lee," said Kean. "I have a hard time getting it up with my wife. She tries, but I don't feel it with her sometimes. It sucks."

Lee looked up at Kean and nodded. "It does suck. Makes me feel like less of a man," Lee continued.

The room was quiet. Lee, the strongest, biggest, and most athletic guy in the room, was cashing in some of his "masculine capital" to share his shame and vulnerability. To his surprise, no one was piling on or joking.

"Lee, I don't see you as any less of anything," said Carlton. "I totally look up to you as a model of what a strong, ethical, honest brother is. You are just taking it to another high level, sharing what you have."

There were nods around the room. This was a significant disclosure for Lee and opened the door for other group members to share more vulnerable material. Carlton, who holds Lee in high esteem, took the floor in his wake.

"I don't want to change the subject, but I am struggling too. My brother made this easier for me to say," Carlton continued. "As you guys can see, I am not small. I love food, the richer and the more flavor the better. If there were no health consequences, I would eat as much as I could. It soothes me. In my fantasy, I might be a world-famous chef. Of course, I'd have to go to culinary school."

"Why not, Carlton?" asked Michael. "You should definitely do that."

"I don't have the academic chops and all the discipline it takes like you, Michael."

"I challenge you on that. If you are interested and motivated, you can learn. I've seen it in many students who find something they are passionate about, and then they take off and follow their dream."

"Wow. I didn't expect that from you." Carlton laughed. "I'm a dreamer, but not much on the follow-through. I should have gone back to school years ago. I am so out of it right now."

"Those sound like excuses, my friend," interjected Peter.

"I'm with Peter on this. You are more than capable, Carlton," added Michael, who seemed to relish having something positive to offer Carlton.

"I probably shouldn't be around food anyway. I lost 50 pounds last summer, and most of it is back on," he replied. He was backpedaling. The guys had good intentions, but I could see Carlton retreating to his shame spot. I needed to intervene.

"Carlton, what does it stir up for you when the guys say they believe in you?" I asked.

"Doc, it doesn't feel real. I want to believe them, but I am still who I am."

"Which is who?"

"I am the guy who will start something but can't finish it. So why should I put effort in when I know it isn't going to work?" Carlton put his hands up and shrugged.

"What's your alternative?" I asked.

"To keep going the way I have been."

"How is that working for you?" I continued.

"I know. You are right. I am going to need some help with this."

"That is why we are here," interjected Ray. Others in the group nodded. Justin and Lee added their support with a spontaneous chorus of "We got your back, man."

Carlton smiled uncomfortably. "I hope I don't let you guys down."

"Do this for you, not us," said Lee. "This is your life, man. We are rooting for you."

"To be honest, the last time I felt this kind of support was back in high school on the football team. I appreciate it. I'll do what I can, homies, but no promises."

"No pressure from us. Just know we support you," replied Kevin.

"Peter, what about you? Where is your passion?" asked Tony, who seemed curious about Peter's background.

"Good question. If you can believe this, I have always been gung ho about religion. I was the poster boy for Christ! Can't say I feel that now, though, but I haven't really found anything that gets me anywhere near the high I used to get," said Peter.

"We have some of that in common," replied Tony. "I was a regular at the Catholic Church in the neighborhood. I found some peace there. I've avoided it lately, especially since I have overtly made the move to leave my wife. Not easy."

"But what do you find passion in?" asked Ray, looking directly at Tony.

"I guess I get caught up in my work. I can diagnose any car problem, do a spiffy tune-up. . . . I fantasize a lot about how to make my business better. In fact, that has always been my escape."

"I'm going to take a risk," said Peter abruptly, seemingly still thinking about his previous answer to Tony. The guys sitting across from him stopped and gave him their full attention. "I haven't been able to admit this to anyone, but I trust you guys." Peter paused. "I fantasize about women. I was pretty content with my life before the accident, but now I have been secretly lusting."

"Welcome to the club," said Neil, a smile on his face.

"Maybe that is a good thing," added Michael.

"I worry it is not a good thing, like I am some kind of sex weirdo. Lust was never something I saw as very Christ-like."

"I know this is a big deal for you, Peter. I haven't told anyone in this group about some of the stuff I have done in my life, so I appreciate your trust. This is hard for me to admit too," said Tony, who seemed to take the cue to go a bit deeper with his disclosure.

"What is making you hesitate?" I asked, knowing that religious guilt was playing into the shame that both Peter and Tony were feeling.

"I've been very secretive. It goes against how I was raised. Sinful," Tony stated. Peter was nodding his head. "I think I should just say it," Tony continued. "I've learned it's better to release my dark thoughts than stress about keeping them in." There was a pause of a few seconds before he continued. "I have been a regular at strip clubs most of my life. I still go occasionally. I'm working on figuring out why I feel compelled, but it's definitely an issue for me."

"Just you saying it makes me feel a little less embarrassed. I want to be a good man, but this feels, I don't know, kind of wrong," added Peter.

"Well, when I have talked to our esteemed leader about this individually, we tossed around the idea that each of us has a 'shadow' self that doesn't necessarily follow all the nice social rules. The more I try to befriend it, the less shame I tend to feel," replied Tony.

"I was hoping we would talk about his," interjected Carlton. "I feel like my whole life has been lived in the shadows. Very little of what I share with people lets them see this part of me. Obviously, my weight is probably a give-away. All I really want them to do is stay at a distance. My weight in itself is probably enough to push them away."

The conversation dropped down into talking about shame, with Carlton, Tony, and Peter helping one another begin to explore this treacherous territory.

"But what are you hiding?" asked Ray.

"Everything. If I let you see what is behind this front, you would be covered in all of my crap. You will see that I am a loser who can't do anything right," replied Carlton.

"Wow. That seems pretty harsh. I don't see you that way," Ray continued.

"That's because I don't show you much. I let you see the 'hip, cool' Carlton mask, not the toilet bowl Carlton who hasn't been able to flush it in years." He picked up a pillow and put it in front of his face so he didn't have to look out. I was aware that I needed to intervene to help Carlton either find some equilibrium or move deeper into his shame so he could work on it. I felt as if the support was there for an intervention.

"Carlton, would you be willing to try something?" I asked.

"I guess," he said, muffled by the large pillow.

"Okay, I'm going to ask you to lie down on your back and let the guys pile pillows on top of you. Is that all right?"

"I guess."

The rest of the group members placed the big square pillows all over Carlton's large body. He lay passively but allowed them to cover him so that from the outside he looked only like a pile of pillows. The pillows were a symbolic manifestation of his defenses. By feeling them protecting him, he might be able to speak more honestly about the inside.

"How does that feel?" I asked.

There was some space near his face so he could breathe and speak. "I like it. I feel protected and safe," he said.

"Good. Can you talk to the group about what it is like to be you on the inside?"

There was some silence. The group members were huddled fairly close around Carlton's buried torso, attentive and curious.

"I feel small. I feel like I have buried myself with crap. If I try anything, I know it will fail, so I hide under here. If I don't try, I won't be hurt. I just will keep my friendly face smiling, hoping no one looks underneath."

"I want to see the real you," said Kean.

"I can't," Carlton responded, sounding almost like a child.

"Why not? You don't trust us?"

"No. I don't trust me. I might have to see what is really there."

"Carlton, see if you can feel the energy of the boy deep down inside. I wonder if you are just trying to protect him from being hurt," I said.

A few seconds of silence followed. "Maybe. I think I had to shut down when my dad died."

"Say more about what you remember about your dad and how you felt when he was around," I responded.

"I felt loved. I felt protected. I didn't worry so much. When he died, everything changed. No one knew how to act. As a family, we just tried to keep going on, but it was all so different. I think I became more self-conscious and less comfortable with who I am. Now look at me, a 350-pound loser."

"You did lose your dad at a crucial point in your life. I want you to try to stay with that boy who lost his dad. What is he feeling?"

Carlton took a few minutes before responding to what seemed like an eternal silence. The men stared at the breathing pile of pillows.

"Scared. I wanted to be held, but I was told I had to man up and not cry. Feels good under the pillows, like being held."

"Good. Stay with that feeling of being protected." The pile of pillows moved up and down with his breathing. "When you feel ready, sit up and push away the pillows."

Slowly Carlton emerged, the pillows falling off him. His face was wet, especially around his eyes. Some of it might have been sweat, but it was also tears. He looked around like a baby bird hatching from an egg. The guys intuitively gave him eye contact and smiles.

"I feel like I am welcome here. I'm not sure I ever really acknowledged that before," Carlton said in a soft voice. He cracked a smile. His face looked softer. "It feels good. Can I take you guys home with me? I'm afraid that when I walk out that door, my shame cloud will be waiting for me. Right now, it is hiding. Feels refreshing."

"Enjoy the feeling. You probably need to practice going to this place to get reacquainted with the inner self that lies beneath the protection," I said. The group formed a circle, arms over one another's shoulders, and made some eye contact.

"I know that took a lot of time, but I appreciate your support," said Carlton with a sincerity that I had not yet seen him show in the group. The guys nodded before breaking the huddle, preparing to return to their lives outside the group room.

## Commentary

The movement of the group from an innocuous prompt about passion led to some powerful psychological work around intimate relationships and shame. The increased trust and cohesion allowed group members to share more deeply but also to react, question, and interact on a more intimate interpersonal level. The mojo discussion got the men in touch with very boylike feelings of engagement while reminding them of what gets in their way. Lee's disclosure about his sexual performance issues with his wife opened the door for other members to go deeper, sharing the shame-based activities in which they were engaged. This also led to acknowledgment of the shadow material, which several of the men were beginning to acknowledge as outlets in their own lives, especially those with strong moral values. Intuitively, I saw an opportunity with Carlton to let him experience some of his shame in the group, with the protection and comfort of the pillows. He was able to talk from the position of his child-self and take in the support of the men, who witnessed his inner dialog. This session also well represented the working stage of group, where each man has the potential to take an issue he is struggling with deeper, knowing the group will support his movement.

### Practical Tips

- Although introducing topics for discussion is helpful in terms of focusing group conversation, it is important to follow the themes that emerge, especially those that are difficult to share, such as intimacy and shame. The flexibility to veer away from the structured activity allowed the group session to go into a more relevant and emotionally valuable direction.
- As a facilitator, it is important to notice the subtle nonverbal behaviors that might indicate tension and conflict between individuals. Even if not addressed immediately, these relationship rifts will need to be confronted at some point in the near future of the group. Not addressing them might lead to the group becoming more hesitant and unsure whether the environment is safe.
- Deep disclosure often begets further disclosures from others. At this stage of the group process, where basic inclusion needs have been established, a member's sharing of difficult material draws others in. This leads to both support and deeper personal responses. Several men were able to approach issues around shame that they had not previously felt comfortable revealing.

## EXPLORING LOSS

Tony opened up one of our February 2017 meetings: "I am really not doing great," he said. "I filed the damn papers for the divorce today, and I thought it would be freeing, but it doesn't feel that way." At this stage of our group, there is less need for a structured prompt. The men know that if something is present, they are free to bring it up as the group begins.

"That's awesome, Tony. I know you have been talking about doing this for a while and couldn't pull the trigger," replied Peter, oblivious to the ambivalence Tony expressed in his voice.

"Listen to me. I am not feeling awesome. I feel like shit. I feel pissed," opined Tony.

"Pissed at who?" I asked, sensing his discomfort.

"Pissed at myself. I should have been able to make it work somehow," Tony replied, the reality of his divorce hitting him and reigniting his guilt.

"But you did it. I know that I have been contemplating leaving my marriage but haven't had the guts to do it," Kean injected. "At least you are moving forward. I am stuck."

"Don't you ever feel like you should have taken care of things? Even though I know that there have been long-standing problems, I can't let go of the feeling of being responsible for the mess and the pain I am causing my wife, kids, and my parents," replied Tony.

"You were all gung ho last time you talked about this. I don't get it," said Peter.

"I think I get it," injected Michael. "As most of you know, I lost a lot of my identity this year. I got fired from being the dean, my mom died, and my wife called it quits. I believe that I could have done something if I was on top of things, or at least it feels like I could have at least saved my job and my marriage."

"Exactly," said Tony. "It's like, what kind of man am I that can't hold my life together?"

"I see it different," injected Ray. "Both of you guys seem like you are trying to live up to some superhero ideal. You both want to take responsibility for things that were outside your control. When I found out I had cancer, I did the same fucking thing. I blamed myself, my lifestyle, and my stupidity. It has taken me a long time to realize that I got cancer. It stinks. Life is not fair. I have to live with my reality. It is uncomfortable, and even if I was some kind of superhero, I wouldn't be able to do anything about it."

"That's what it has been like with my mom. She keeps coming back from the edge of death with her cancer. I want to help her, but all I can do is be there. I don't like to think about it," added Justin, who had been observing but not participating in the last few sessions.

"So, Tony, you are angry about the situation, but you also are not talking about the loss that comes with taking action. You seem to want to be able to act without feeling the pain," I said. Out of the corner of my eye, I could see that Peter was now looking down. His facade of positivity seemed to vanish. My attention shifted.

"Peter, what's going on for you?" I asked. Peter looked up, eyes glassy. He wiped a tear with his hand. "This discussion is really touching me. I really feel like I still blame myself in many ways for the deaths of my wife and child."

"Come on, man. That is not true. You didn't do it," injected Neil.

"Neil, I appreciate your support of Peter, but he needs to feel this. It is part of his healing process," I intervened, knowing that the tears represented a breakthrough for Peter, who only shed his tears in private.

"I know intellectually I couldn't do anything, but it is hard not to feel super responsible. The voice inside says, 'I didn't do enough to save them,'" replied Peter.

"That part of you doesn't want to feel powerless," I proposed.

"No. I just go numb when I try to accept what happened as an accident and not mine or God's fault. The pain is leaking out of me right now, but I can't go any further," he added. Tony moved next to Peter and put his massive arm around his shoulder.

"It's okay to feel it," shared Tony. "You are helping me acknowledge the pain I feel in breaking up my family. I can't imagine losing them permanently, but I know you are feeling like you abandoned them underneath. We are here to support you. Believe it."

Peter looked up at the group, his cheeks moist. A wounded animal sound wailed from him. The sound continued, muffled, with his head buried in Tony's chest. I could also see that Tony's eyes were watery. The rest of the group closed in to form a tighter circle.

"Man, we just need to be here for each other," said Ray from the circle.

"It's okay to feel it," added Michael, who seemed more engaged with the grief as he saw it in some of the other men.

Justin, who usually presented the poker face, even when he was talking personally, was flushed and a bit teary-eyed.

"I always thought crying was weak, but this feels gutsy and strong," said Kevin, who had his arms around both Kean and Lee. There were nods around the hug circle.

## Commentary

The group seemed to collectively become a container for both guilt and grief. There was a sense that some of the loss experienced could have been prevented or averted. We were all feeling the deep sadness, as if all the losses each of us had experienced were being summoned into the room. We were crying for one another and for ourselves. There was no rationalizing or explaining. The looks we were giving one another were enough to say this is good and right.

Men typically don't cry much, and especially not around each other. No one ever really gets over loss; rather, it hangs around in the recesses of consciousness. It may find a venue in dreams or when reminded by a situation or memory. The best any of us can do is to give the grief space to be expressed. In day-to-day routine life, we often protect ourselves by focusing elsewhere. When we do acknowledge it, there is some protective mechanism in our heads that wants us to feel as if we could have done something, maybe we had some control. This is what haunts us, reminding us that if something different could have occurred, we might not be experiencing this pain. We try to rewrite history to produce a new outcome. Once we acknowledge that it can't be done, the pain strikes hard again, but in the container of the group, we can stay with it a little longer.

The group is at a stage where even the most traditionally masculine men are willing to share some of their vulnerability. The feeling of sadness, loss of control, and psychological pain lingered, leaving everyone in the room without their main defenses. The mutual support, both verbal and physical, allowed several men to touch their grief and experience themselves as emotional beings. Peter and Ray, further along in accepting loss as a part of their lives, assist Tony, Michael, and Justin in staying connected to their feelings. My role was to facilitate "being" with the sadness rather than intellectualizing or diminishing its significance.

### Practical Tips

- It is important to value the expression of feeling, especially at this stage of the group. Loss is a common experience. One man's loss may easily trigger others' reexperiencing or even surfacing feelings of deep sadness. The feeling of guilt often accompanies loss as a means to feel some control.
- In the middle stages of the men's group, I have noticed that the members are more likely to work off each other. One man's sharing often is a catalyst for others to feel, speak, and feel connection to one another's deeper issues.
- The facilitator stills needs to bring the concerns that have occurred outside the group into the here and now. Otherwise, the group can regress into monologues that other members listen to passively. In this session, it was important to encourage personal reactions and sharing in response to the initial comments of guilt introduced by the initiator of the discussion.

## THE CAMPOUT

The fire from our March 2017 annual men's group camping trip could probably be seen from space. Our parked cars and trucks circled the rogue campsite outside of Joshua Tree National Park, at least a half mile from any other campers. One of Tony's business associates who owned a lumberyard had let him pile his pickup full of enough scrap wood to burn for days. I had brought old African drums and other percussion instruments. After cooking burgers and hot dogs on a grill, the drumming began. At first the sound was like random taps, but soon there was a definite heartbeat rhythm. Each man found his own movement that blended into waves of primitive sound. It was as if we were back in time, a hunting party in a wild place far from home. Several of the guys had never camped out, so those who had acted as guides and mentors.

Justin, who usually played it cool, was like a little kid looking under the tree on Christmas morning. He had pushed us to hike through a big canyon during the day, where we found a desert oasis. He had taken off his shirt and was now dancing around the fire. Ray, his gray ponytail swinging from side to side in beat with the drums, smiled as he watched the youngest member of the group lose his inhibition.

"Make it rain, Justin!" he whooped over the drums.

The giant full moon came up over the Chocolate Mountains, grabbing everyone's attention. Each man was bathed in a celestial glow. The drumming slowed.

"I've done my share of partying, but I never celebrated the moon coming up like this," said Carlton, who was substance free for almost three months. "The natural high!" He laughed.

"This is the closest the moon will be to Earth for the next 33 years. It is truly a magnificent phenomenon. We should be able to see some of those craters with detail," announced Michael as he worked on his portable telescope setup. This is what I had hoped would happen out here in the desert. Talking through problems is one thing, but getting some extra assistance from this surreal desert environment gets to all of the senses. Over the years the spring campout had been a way to apply the learning in a new setting. Extended time together allowed for more natural interactions that reflected our accumulated intimacy.

Car headlights and dust moved toward us. I hoped it was our missing group member, Neil, who had been doing something he couldn't miss, or so he said. The late-model Mercedes bounced over the rutted dirt road before stopping at the site.

"Neil. You made it!" cried out Kean, his closest friend in the group. Neil, with a white collared shirt, designer jeans, and black dress shoes, looked a bit unprepared for the wilderness.

"Glad you could fit us into your busy schedule," said Kevin, with a bit of sarcasm.

"Would never miss this. Where are the strippers?" he retorted as he moved toward the fire circle.

"You would say that, Neil. Did your girlfriend decide to let you leave her side for a few hours?" replied Kevin, cutting straight to Neil's weakness.

"Leave him alone, Kevin. He made it. That's what is important," said Kean, handing Kevin a tambourine. "You eat?"

"Yeah. Not sure I can stay the night. Got early-morning clinic. Besides that, I didn't bring a sleeping bag or any of that stuff."

"I guess it's a myth that doctors are always prepared," responded Kevin.

"Don't worry, Kevin. I do have the emergency medical kit in the trunk if you need it."

"Why are you busting his balls so hard, Kevin?" asked Kean, who seemed to pick up on the rising tension that Kevin's comments were fueling.

Kevin waved him off and then looked at me. "Doc, we are still officially in group out here, right?"

"Sure. Anything you would say in group is fair game out here," I responded, wondering what was coming next but also wanting the guys to apply the intimacy of our group sessions.

"Neil, I feel like you are not being very real with us. It's bullshit that you show up here like you are making a guest appearance rather than committing to being with the group," said Kevin in a serious tone that jolted the casualness of the camping atmosphere.

The drumming stopped. The only sound was the crackle of the fire.

"What do you want me to say, Kevin?" Neil replied.

"The truth. I have a good bullshit detector. I think you are scared to be real with us. You were on a fucking date even though we had all agreed to be on the campout."

Neil looked at me for a signal. I shrugged, not sure what to say. I knew that this interpersonal conflict had been building. I wasn't quite prepared in the moment.

Michael, who had been quiet most of the night, jumped into the fray.

"At least he has a girlfriend, Kevin. This isn't a cult. He is free to do what he wants. Hell, if I had a girlfriend, I might blow this off," he said with an assertiveness that I hadn't heard before in my interactions with him.

"Really? I get you defending Neil, Michael. You've been coming to group regularly and have shared your pain. I respect what you say, but Neil has been doing this crap for a while."

Neil's face was lit crimson by the fire. He looked hurt. I felt a need to intervene. Kevin was steaming. As much as I enjoyed the campout as a regular guy, I had a role to play.

"Kevin, you seem really pissed off. What is Neil triggering for you?" I asked.

"I don't know. I just hate it when he skates around the truth. He's not being real."

"Say more," I said with conviction.

"I have worked hard to trust people in this group, and to be honest, I don't trust him."

"Say it directly to Neil." He looked at Neil, who hadn't moved. Half of Kevin's face was shadowed, and the other side glowed orangey red from the fire.

"Neil, I don't trust you. You don't have my back. That's important to me if we are going to have a meaningful, deep experience in this group."

"Why is this so strong for you, Kevin? Maybe I'm more superficial than you, but I do care about this group," replied Neil.

"You say you care, but you remind me of all the people in my life who have said they were there for me, but when push came to shove they weren't."

"This isn't about you, Kevin. I live this way. I never commit fully. I am always looking for the next shiny thing, even in women. Especially women," Neil said with clarity.

"Why don't you work on that a little fucking harder? Shit, I am working my ass off to be able to trust people and it is not easy."

"I didn't know I mattered that much to you," replied Neil. "You usually roll your eyes when I am telling stories about my relationships. I thought you were bored."

"Not bored. Just want you to stop the stupid cycle you are in. It seems so easy to see your issues. You don't really trust women either to be there for you. I get that," said Kevin.

"You get me, Kevin? Then why not give me support? All I get is contempt." Below his breath Neil then added, "Asshole."

"What did you say, Neil?" asked Kevin.

"Nothing," he replied.

"I can be an asshole, but at least I give a shit enough to express it," Kevin responded.

"Why are you all over me? I was in a good mood and ready to be here with the guys. Now I feel like I've been brought before the Spanish Inquisition," Neil replied.

There was a pause before Kevin softened, his breathing more pronounced. "I think I'm jealous. I have been betrayed too much to even try to go out on dates. You go out as if it doesn't fucking matter. But I think I finally understand it. You don't trust them enough to be impacted by betrayal. I wish I could do that, but I can sense betrayal even before it happens. That's my fucking fatal flaw."

"You actually are not that different from Neil. You both are protecting your vulnerability," I interjected.

Kevin nodded. The storm that had risen in him was now gone. Kevin's shadow, cast from the fire, stretched toward Neil, who spontaneously moved toward Kevin with open arms.

"I hear you, brother," said Neil as he moved in to hug Kevin. I flinched, not sure how Kevin would receive the gesture. Michael started banging on his big drum. The rest of the group followed with rapid, applause-like drumming. Kevin reacted to the beat by opening himself to Neil's hug. Smiles appeared on their faces. "That's how we get through interpersonal conflict," I thought to myself. It's dangerous but worth the risk. I remembered why I've been doing this for 35 years.

## Commentary

Over the years, the weekend campout has been a way for the men to bring into the group the aspects of themselves that normally are not seen. Encountering the members outside of the group room in a rugged setting allows for a more "doing" approach to interaction. Whether it is putting up a tent, cutting vegetables, taking a hike, or building a fire, the group joins together to create an interpersonal environment that takes advantage of the relational intimacy that has been built in the weekly meetings. Without the constraints of time or space, the conversation and activity is a bit more organic and retreat-like in its nature, rather than contrived. Although I still am aware of my role as a facilitator, the group also sees me more as the fellow everyday guy in this setting.

Marked by small skirmishes of interaction in the group during the year, the conflict between Kevin and Neil had been building. When Neil showed up late and unprepared for the retreat, it intensified Kevin's built-up resentment. His own history of betrayal and neglect were triggered by Neil's cavalier style and seemingly shallow reflections about his relationships with women. Kevin and Neil both shared a fear of intimacy, but their defense styles clashed. Kevin withdrew and harbored his anger just beneath the surface. Neil tended to rely on superficial conversation to defend against his fears. The fight was good for both of them, especially as it played out in the circle of the group members, who had some percussion instruments available to express what they were feeling. This seemed to enhance the encounter and give it added significance. There was relief when both Kevin and Neil backed off from physical violence and instead acknowledged the common intimacy fear they shared. I hoped that this would open up their relationship, as each had important feedback and information for the other.

### Practical Tips

- The campout weekend is a unique aspect to our group process. Although some practitioners employ an extended workshop model (see Englar-Carlson & Stevens, 2014), it typically is not combined with a weekly group format. By having extended time, the members can interact in a more natural setting, employing many of the skills learned in the group. As seen in the interaction between Kevin and Neil, it also is ripe for interpersonal encounters that require the facilitator to be prepared.
- The setting does raise issues around boundaries. Although we are in a protected, safe space with no other campers around, the leader does not have the same office space and time parameters. The group has many more possible interactions, from cooking to sleeping arrangements. The psychological distance between the members and leader is minimal in this environment. This requires the leader to be comfortable with himself and be prepared for members to see aspects of the leader that they have not seen in the more controlled setting.
- The camping environment also raises issues about how much structure to impose. Obviously hikes, meals, and sleeping arrangements must be clarified. But there is also more time for one-on-one and smaller group interactions. Typically, I have had structured activities that allow for extended storytelling, as well as percussion instruments to encourage group bonding by playing together.
- Group members sign waivers to release the leader from liability in this setting. This is typically done with the initial paperwork signed before the men's group begins in the fall.
- The extended camping weekend often leads to more connection and intimacy and typically has a positive impact on in-group relationships.

## RELATIONSHIPS

"I wish I could be happy with 'good enough,' but I am forever pulled toward exciting, intriguing, smart, and beautiful," opined Neil early in one of our April 2017 groups. "I realize I am probably fucked up, but I don't know how to settle."

"I like the idea of exciting. Why do we have to settle?" asked Kean.

"Because it is reality," interjected Kevin with authority.

"Say more, Kevin," I intervened.

"I lived the fantasy, and it was just a fantasy. My ex-wife was as beautiful and intriguing as they come, but she was very flawed. I never wanted to see it. Now I can't help seeing every woman I meet as messed up in some way," he continued.

"I know we have had our differences, so don't take this the wrong way, but I think that is a distortion on your part, Kevin," replied Neil. "Women are flawed, but they are also complicated and as unsure of themselves as we are. What are you expecting them to be?"

"Good question. I grew up without any nurturing from a mother or father. Maybe I just don't know how I am supposed to relate to them in a healthy way. I know I want someone I can trust and who would have my back. Don't know what that feels like."

"My wife has been a saint to put up with me and my depression," added Lee. "She accepts me more than I accept myself. I guess I am fortunate."

"You definitely are," said Tony. "I was married for a long time to someone who wasn't really capable of supporting me. Maybe I didn't let her, but I sensed she couldn't do it. I thought it was my job to take care of her. It wasn't mutual."

"I think my wife was the same," added Michael. "I didn't share much of my emotional life with her, but neither did she. I realize now how avoidant I was of conflict and how out of touch I was with myself. I can't be in another relationship until I am more willing to mix it up and say where I am coming from."

"It seems like we are really talking about a couple of different themes here. One is about what you need from a partner, and the other is about what you are willing to bring into a relationship," I interjected, wanting our discussion to move a bit deeper.

"Well, I think I started this conversation," said Neil. "It's because I realize that I can only go so far in a relationship before I start to sabotage it."

"What do you mean?" asked Ray. I looked around, and everyone in the meeting seemed engaged with this topic.

"I am really good at making a woman feel like I am into them, which I am, but then I don't know how to deepen the relationship. I just want to have sex and hang out. I don't actually want to know about their problems and flaws. I idealize them. But then, we don't have much to talk about after a while," Neil added.

"That is fucked up, Neil. What are you afraid of?" asked Kean.

"Like I said before, I don't think I can sustain a real relationship."

"You did with your wife for many years," retorted Kean.

"Yes, and then I realized there was more to a relationship than the practical, but sometimes I wonder if all relationships end up in the practical mode. Once you know someone, the mystery and discovery is gone."

"You seem addicted to the rush of a new relationship," interjected Carlton. "I know addiction, and what you describe sounds like the beginning of a new drug."

"I know that is probably true, but I can't unhook myself," Neil replied.

"You don't want to. Admit it, Neil," said Kevin.

Neil looked deflated. He dropped his head, as if he was peering inward. I wondered if something had broken through. Most of the time, guys are pretty supportive of the pursuit of a potential partner, even if it is a vicarious thrill. At this stage of the group, the members seem to care enough about Neil to not go there. Instead they are challenging him. The previous encounters with Kevin, especially when they faced off at the campout, had cracked an opening. They triggered each other, and here it was again. The peer feedback seemed to be more impactful than I could be with my interventions in individual therapy. Neil was staring at an emotional abyss of inner emptiness that sat beneath his womanizing behavior. The room was quiet until he broke the silence.

"I don't know what to do, guys. If I don't have a woman in my life, it feels empty. Take that away from me and I am just plain old Dr. Neil, an aging physician who is surviving life, not drinking it in."

"Neil, can you just stay with that feeling for a minute? It is important to know what lies underneath. Say more about what's down there," I intervened, sensing his vulnerability.

Neil's face had a blank look. His eyes seemed to be defocused but moist. He hesitated and then put his hand on his forehead. "I am afraid."

"Afraid of what?" I asked, knowing that I was at the portal to his depth.

"My depression. I'm afraid I won't be able to move beyond it. That is what I hide." He shook his head as if something from his past was creeping into his consciousness.

"What is it?" I asked.

"As a boy, I used to feel this way a lot. I became a really good student, burying myself with homework when everyone else was probably out playing. I fantasized about great things I was going to do when I got older, but in reality I sat in my room, feeling lonely and depressed." As he spoke, Kean and Peter moved next to Neil and put their hands on the back of his shoulders. At first he tensed at the show of support, but then he seemed to relax into it.

"It's okay to feel your pain," said Peter, his eyes glassy.

"We have your back. You can be real here," added Kean. From across the room, Kevin met Neil's gaze. "I think this is the first time I have seen the real you, Neil. Believe it or not, I can relate to you. You are brave. I'm not sure I could share that, but I feel it too."

## Commentary

Neil was one of the last group members to break into his depth. Previous groups in which several of the men shared their pain and grief had not penetrated him very deeply, but the confrontation at the campout had lowered the walls of his psychological "fortress." For the group to proceed at a more intimate level, it needed him to drop down and face himself, something he had resisted up until now. The continued push from Kevin, who was also working off of Neil's character style, kept some pressure on. When his outer shell finally broke, we all got to see a deeper view of Neil, one that was vulnerable and in pain. In the process he got some of the validation and support he usually sought from the women he pursued.

The theme of what each of us brings to relationships is an important one in a men's group. It is easy to blame others for failing relationship connections. This session showed some willingness to own what each man brings into the relationship. Tony, Kevin, and Michael were able to articulate more about their own needs and not blame their partners but realize that they contributed to the relationship dynamics. This session exemplified the continuous exploration of how the interpersonal dynamics were playing out in the group setting and its impact on individual growth.

## Practical Tips

- Although it may seem that there is not enough time in a given session to work through the concerns of members, group depth builds on work in previous sessions, leading to more openness and authentic sharing. The breakthrough by Neil had its beginnings in earlier group interactions.
- The shifting alliances in the group often reflect how close various members are feeling to one another. By paying attention to the subgroups and interaction patterns, it is possible to track the group process. This helps a leader make decisions about whether a particular topic or issue is most relevant in the present. The topic of relationships seemed important given that several of the members were struggling with intimacy and willing to take responsibility for their parts in past failures.
- Bringing Neil's struggle into the present allowed other members to relate to him and give him positive feedback for sharing vulnerability. It was particularly powerful to hear Kevin praise Neil for his realness, given their ongoing interpersonal conflict.

# 12

# Integrating Learning and Letting Go

## *Scenes From the Later Stage of the Men's Group*

In the later stages of Deepening group psychotherapy, men are often more comfortable speaking up about what they need from others. They can be more vocal about this because, in addition to developing trust, they have learned—mainly from one another—the vocabulary to fit their struggles and some tools for working through those struggles.

### THE RUT

In May 2017, it was time to start thinking ahead about what the conclusion of the men's group would look like. "Given we are getting into the final 2 months of the group, is there anything anyone wants to share or work on? Maybe something you have been putting off talking about here?" I opened. There was silence, some body movements, and blank stares, but I anticipated that a few of the guys who had not spoken much recently would volunteer to take the risk to share.

"I don't want to bring this up, but I know that because I don't want to I probably should," replied Kean, who had been helpful with others in the group but rarely took time for himself to share his inner conflict.

"It's okay. Take your time. We are here for you, brother," interjected Ray, who had really embraced the group as his family.

http://dx.doi.org/10.1037/0000132-013
*Deepening Group Psychotherapy With Men: Stories and Insights for the Journey,*
by F. E. Rabinowitz

"I am feeling stuck, like I am in a rut. I come in here every week and realize I have intellectual insight and empathy for others, but I don't do anything to change my situation."

"What do you mean?" asked Justin.

"I know you guys feel like you know me, but there are things I haven't talked about. I want to trust everyone, and I do on some core level, but I have some skeletons in my closet that I haven't shared with anyone except maybe Fred." Kean looked over at me. I nodded, giving him some nonverbal encouragement.

"This is really hard for me. When you guys were talking about women the other week, I realized that I am pretty confused about the whole relationship thing."

"That is pretty vague," commented Kevin.

"I know, but it is complicated. You guys are not that judgmental, but this is delicate for me." Kean paused for a few seconds, then took a deep breath and blurted out, "I think I might be gay or bi or something in that spectrum. There, I said it." He looked down, not making eye contact.

"Wow," countered Ray, not realizing he was saying it out loud. Quickly, he added, "That's cool, Kean. To each his own. Not a problem for me."

"What makes you think you're gay, Kean? You are married to a woman. I'm not judging, but I don't get it," said Peter.

"I wish I got it," replied Kean. "I've had some experiences with guys that made me question my sexuality. When I was young, I experimented, and maybe that is something I need to look at. Maybe that conditioned me. I don't know. I have held this in for so many years. I felt like I was being dishonest with you guys by not talking about it."

There was silence in the room. Kean looked down, still unwilling to make eye contact. Carlton interjected, "Just so you know, Kean, I've had some experiences when I was younger with guys. I don't think it is that uncommon."

"Me too," added Ray. "I was in some funky orgies during my hippie commune days, and it got going with both guys and girls."

"I was molested by an older guy on my football team. I've never told anybody," said Lee, without expression. The room again became silent. Kean looked up at the three men who shared their revelations.

"Shit. That blows me away. I thought I was just a freak. I wish I had known that about you guys. Maybe I wouldn't have been so frightened to bring it up," replied Kean.

"Your bringing it up lets us share some of our secrets. I would have never mentioned it if you hadn't had the courage to talk about it," replied Lee.

"Before I share any more, is anyone not okay with this?" asked Kean.

"Kean, is there anyone you are worried will judge you in here?" I asked.

"No. I don't think so."

"Then why are you asking? Look around the room and address who you might fear will be judgmental," I offered, sensing Kean's fear of being too exposed.

"This is hard," he responded as he carefully scanned the room. "I wonder about you, Peter. I know you have been a hard-core Christian and might not be okay with the whole gay thing."

Peter nodded and said, "I know I was raised in a pretty judgmental tradition, but I've gotten to know you in here, and honestly, I want you to share whatever you want. It's hard for me to wrap my head around it personally, but I am no one to talk about sinning. I haven't been interested in guys in that way, but I believe we are all God's children. Since the deaths of my wife and daughter, I have been humbled. We all have our burdens to work out here. You haven't lost anything in my eyes."

"Thanks for saying that, Peter. I appreciate your support," said Kean, still looking tense.

"Anyone else you are worried about judging you?" I asked.

"Tony. What about you? You have strong opinions and that Catholic upbringing."

"Kean, you are my friend. I have nothing but respect for you. I am like Peter. I wouldn't probably experiment myself, but I don't have a problem with you working this out in here. I know you as Kean, not by any one quality or label," replied Tony.

"I appreciate that," answered Kean.

"Anyone else you worried about?" I asked.

"Myself. I'm probably the one who is not okay with all of this. I can feel myself going numb, like it is surreal that I am talking about it. I am outside my body looking in. It's been a secret part of me for so long."

"You only have to go as far as you want, Kean. You know this is a process," I reassured him.

"I know. I feel like I am betraying my wife and my kids by even sharing it in here. They don't know, and now you guys do. This group knows more about me that anyone in my family."

"We are brothers, Kean. It is safe here," added Ray.

"I don't know if this will help you with sharing, but you know I cheated on my wife from the start of our marriage. I used to sneak out of the house in the middle of the night and hit the strip club. Not very Catholic of me," shared Tony in a serious tone.

"Tell us about the conflict, Kean. You've been carrying it around for a while," said Lee. "We all have our demons."

Kean hesitated before responding to Lee. "I don't like being the focus of attention. I think it was enough for me to share that lifelong demon right now. I don't feel ready to do much more. Thanks for the support, guys. I know I can bring it up now, and I will when I am ready. I need to. I don't want to be phony here, and sometimes I have been," Kean replied, eager to get the spotlight off him.

"Why not now?" asked Michael, who had been quiet up to this point.

"Just not ready," he replied.

"Michael, is there anything that Kean's revelation stirred up in you?" I asked. I had a sense that Michael was hoping to watch Kean work in a voyeuristic way. He needed a model for how to work through difficult emotional material. Maybe this was an opportunity for him to work in the group.

"I have been questioning myself a lot about what I want. I have played it safe my whole life, you know, staying in my head. I say I want to be more in touch with my emotions, but I feel like I don't do anything that different. I still read, think about logical solutions, but I really don't spend much time in my gut."

"Is there something on your mind that you think would be good to work on here?" I asked. Michael seemed to go straight to his head, tilting it sideways and looking up. "I don't know how important this is, but it popped into my mind. When Kean talked about his sexuality, it made me think about my own. I was a virgin before I got married, and my wife was the only woman I have ever been with. I don't think I am very sexual. The opportunities don't present themselves. I wonder if I am asexual?"

"What kind of porn do you look at?" asked Justin bluntly.

"To be honest, I am not one to consume porn. I'm not that interested in seeing actors pretending to have fun having sex. I can't identify with them. I wonder if I am blocking my sexual response the same as I block my emotions? I know I must sound really naive, but this whole conversation has stirred up my lack of sex drive and what that potentially means about me as a man."

"Michael, I'm not sure how to respond to you. I don't know if I should just be supportive or confront you to go further. You've shared information that is pretty intense, but I really can't get a read on how you really feel about it," replied Kevin.

"Yes, I think we would all like to help you, Michael. My opinion is you just need some more experience with different people to get a feel for it," said Lee.

"We don't need to fix Michael right now. It is wonderful that he is feeling comfortable enough to open up what is going on inside of him," I intervened, worried that the group dialog was going to lead to a list of suggestions Michael should try. This seemed premature, given he was just beginning to share some of his inner experience, not just his intellect, with the group.

Without showing any signs of embarrassment, Michael replied, "Maybe I'm skipping steps here. I have only dated one person in my life, so just going out with someone on a date would be a big deal. The sex part seems further away,"

"What stops you from going out?" asked Justin, who seemed to not believe what he was hearing from Michael.

"Justin, I am so used to being alone, I don't really pursue it. It is easier to just read and work and ignore that part of my life."

"It's a rut so deep you don't know even know you are in it," said Kean, who seemed to perk up hearing the other men respond to Michael's lack of dating and sexual experience.

"Yes. I guess you could say that," replied Michael.

"I'm realizing that as long as you put off what you know you need to deal with, the deeper the rut gets. I guess the first step is acknowledging being stuck," added Kean, who seemed to use Michael's revelations to further his own process.

"I'm with you on that. I am okay if you guys push me. I need it," said Michael.

Almost in unison, the several group members responded back, "We will push you."

### Commentary

The group feels safe enough for Kean and Michael to talk about their sexuality, even though it deviates from the traditional masculine norms. The pressure on Kean to share more of himself was a result of the intimacy of the group at this stage. He felt as if he was not being a good friend or group member if he didn't share some of his deeper conflicts. The sharing is a relief but not a solution for Kean. The importance of the emotional support and the sharing of some of the members' sexual experiences takes away some of his shame. By confronting his own fears of judgment, he allowed himself to move toward work on the issue in the future. Michael's admission that he had very little sexual drive or experience was a big risk on his part. It allowed him to show his vulnerability while receiving support from the group.

As the group moves toward ending for the year, I pushed to make sure that difficult concerns were not put off. Although not everyone will get closure, it would be worse to not bring up issues that were significant to the individuals in the group. The other dynamic that was illustrated in this scene was how the group members helped out one another. Among the men, there was a sense of agency that they could not only share deep, personal material but also be therapeutic in their feedback to one another.

### Practical Tips

- As the end date for group approaches, it is important to remind the members that the experience will not last forever. This time pressure to work on unfinished issues can be helpful to those who have hesitated to share deeper concerns. Even though members can recommit to be a part of the group in the future, the coming 3-month hiatus still represents an ending.

- At this stage, group members can handle more direct confrontations from the leader and other members. The leverage of the group coming to an end for the year is often powerful motivation to not leave unfinished issues on the table. At the same time, it is unrealistic to believe that all concerns will be wrapped up neatly.

- The group leader should also do his or her own assessment about what hasn't been discussed and address these concerns directly.

## FEEDBACK, SUPPORT, LETTING GO, AND HOLDING ON

The group takes a 3-month hiatus in July before reconvening in October. The last groups of June represent the end of a 9-month weekly journey. My focus in the final groups is to make sure that the members give and receive feedback. It is also a time of reflection on progress made and direction for the near and long-term future.

"Since we're getting ready for the summer break, and for some of you this is the end of your experience in this group, it might be good to think about what you feel you have accomplished, what you wish you might have worked on but didn't, and to get some honest feedback from the others in the group. We have just a couple of groups left to make this happen, but it's up to each of you to step up to make the most of our time," I stated at the beginning of the group.

"I would like some feedback from the group," said Kevin. "I feel like you guys can see the flimsy foundation my life is really built on. I know I am a cop in the outside world, but I feel almost too exposed in my emotional life."

"What do you mean by too exposed?" asked Peter.

"It's a long story, but I grew up without much in the way of parenting. I learned everything on my own through my encounters with life. I wish I had a more safe, secure upbringing so I would know what that was like. I am always vigilant and on guard. I don't know what I would have become if I had grown up like Michael, with two college professor parents. I love literature, but maybe I could have become a professor or at least believed I was professor material. I did the best I could, but I knew I would never be good enough. I think becoming a cop was my way of doing something on the right side with a skill set I could take from the street," continued Kevin, who clearly had been contemplating his life journey. "So, I guess I should go there, to the broken core of my being. What do you guys think?"

"I think we are all broken in some way," said Ray. "I had the stable father and mother, but the quality of the contact was pretty sketchy. I wonder how much more I could have been if my dad was more around and less judgmental."

"I relate to that too, Ray," added Justin. "My dad is also this doctor who I have never really talked to on a real level. I sometimes imagine how different life would have been for me if he was around. This is hard stuff for me. I need to work on getting the guts to call him and face him. I've avoided it hoping that sometime soon I would be able to do it. But I keep putting it off, and it's never going to happen. That is something I need to set as a priority. I've been a real chickenshit."

"Wow. I see you both as tough dudes," Lee commented, looking at Justin and Kevin. "It must be pretty scary for you to not just take it on. I guess I relate to trying to stay tough, when I should be going the other way. I know my depression is made worse by my attitude of thinking I can do everything by myself, and then when I hurt and fail, I can just blame myself."

"Lee, I wonder if you want any feedback from guys in the group about how they see you," I asked, wondering if Lee's disclosure was perhaps an invitation.

"Yes and no. But given that I am here to learn and grow, I do want feedback. I know, I should ask specifically certain members," Lee continued. "Carlton, I know you've said I am a model for you, but I just want it to be real with us. I want to know how you really see me, not just because I'm a fellow Black man here."

"Lee, I still look up to you. You have been honest and strong, and that has given me hope."

"Anything specific about Lee you can point to, Carlton?" I asked.

"I just like how you carry yourself. You don't brag, and you don't try to be something you're not. I know you were a football star at one point, and I wanted to be that. Seeing you not use that as your identity makes me admire you more. That's the best way I can put it. You show grace and restraint and realness," said Carlton.

"Man, that means a lot coming from you, Carlton. I may act too cool. I need to be a little more emotional and let everyone see a bit more of my inner doubts," replied Lee.

"I relate to you a lot, Lee," injected Tony. "I know we had our differences early in the group about the election and all that, but you are someone whose struggle mirrors mine. I know I walk around with a big energy field and most people just back off. I need to share more of my struggles too. I hope we both continue the group into next year, because I do want to get to know you better."

"I appreciate it, Tony. I was thinking about how worked up I got in the fall, and how pissed I was with you. The more I've listened to you, the more I have respect. I think we are actually pretty similar in our ways of walking the world, especially how others react to our physical size and perceived strength. I am open to getting to know you better too."

"Let's get back to Kevin," I intervened. "You were wanting feedback, and we moved to Ray and Justin in response to your comment about your broken core."

"It's all right. I'm good," replied Kevin

"No. You don't need to take a backseat, Kevin. You are as important as anyone in here," said Peter. "I know I admire your strength and conviction. You've been willing to challenge yourself, and I know it's not comfortable for you."

"Thanks, Peter. I get frustrated. I want to trust, but it is hard when I don't trust myself inside. I'm good at picking up on the bad guys because I know what it feels like to be bad."

"That is heavy, Kevin," commented Neil. "You and I have had our battles, but if there is anyone in this group who has pushed me to become more real, it is you, Kevin. You can see right through me. I tried to ignore it, but it's like you are a walking lie detector. I need that. You don't call me out if you don't care."

"You are right, Neil. I do care. I do see you as being able to get past your bullshit to make a go of relationships. I wouldn't mind having some of that."

"Well, I'll trade you. Give me some of the cop intensity and toughness, and I'll show you how to pick up women," Neil said with a smile. This was not something he could have said months ago.

"He could be your wingman, Kevin," joked Kean.

"Seriously, I think we learned a lot from each other, Neil," Kevin continued. "I really got a lot from all of you in here. It's like having a bunch of different mirrors I can see myself in. My mirrors growing up were so distorted, I felt like I was just getting by. I adapted to my environment. In here, I really appreciate the honest feedback."

"I know I have probably grown more emotionally this year in group than anytime I can remember," interjected Michael, who had a stubble beard and wore a T-shirt and shorts, a far cry from his more uptight, formal appearance when he initially entered the therapeutic arena.

"Anyone in particular you'd like to get some feedback from?" I asked.

"I guess I'd want it from anyone, but I'd like to hear from Tony."

"What is it about Tony that he came to mind first?" I asked.

Michael hesitated a few seconds before speaking. "Tony is strong and direct. If I am honest, I need those qualities to round out my personality. I question whether I have the cojones to make it in this world. Sometimes I feel like I am Sisyphus with the rock on my back trudging endlessly up the mountain and never reaching the top."

"I'm flattered you picked me, Michael. You are the smartest dude I've ever met. It means a lot coming from you," responded Tony.

"Wow. I guess that is good. I want to know what you think I need to do to be more tough or strong," said Michael.

"Michael. You have to be you. You can't be anyone else. You are intelligent. That is strength. Like everyone has been saying in here, you need to listen to what your emotions tell you. Your journey is yours. It certainly isn't mine."

"What are you feeling in response to Tony's comments?" I asked Michael.

"I know he is right. I know I have to take some chances in areas that aren't my strengths. It feels good to be seen on my road, even when I can't really see my destination."

"Damn right, Michael," responded Tony. "You got to see yourself as someone worthy of being seen. You got so much going for you." He then moved toward Michael and gave him a bear hug. The group members watched the two unlikely men embracing. There were nods and smiles.

With only a few minutes left in the group, Carlton spoke. "I want to say something. I know that I have a lot of work to do on myself still, but this group has really given me the energy to stay with my plan. I know that I still need to lose more weight and get myself back to school, but just being able to keep my motivation going is more than I can ever remember. Knowing I face you each week, you guys have kept me accountable. I'm worried that when we are off this summer I won't have the support."

"Maybe some of us can get together over the summer informally," said Ray. "I'd certainly want to continue to meet. I've come to depend on this place where I can just be myself."

"Me too," said Lee. "Carlton, we will make sure that we have each other's backs this summer."

As the group came to a close, the guys stood and formed a circle, arms around one another. "The last group will be at Neil's house for a potluck. You guys can work out what to bring on the listserv. Any last words before we leave tonight?" I asked. I could feel a tightening of the arms around my shoulders. There were some longing looks, with eye contact. No one wanted to break the circle, so we stayed connected for a good 2 minutes before I nodded and the group loosened its grip.

## Commentary

The last stage of group often has mixed agendas. For some of the men, it is about consolidating the learning that has occurred. The difference between what it felt like starting out and how it feels at the end is a barometer of the growth. Even though it is hard to track the subtle changes, knowing the group is coming to an end highlights them. The other issue that often arises is a feeling of loss, a conflict zone issue that men often are uncomfortable addressing. By having developed a deep, trusting relationship with men whom at first he barely knew, each man has some sense of anticipating missing the intimacy of this space each week.

Although many interpersonal dynamics haven't been fully acknowledged or addressed, there is a sense that they could be. The value of receiving feedback from caring "mirrors" allows the men to see themselves differently. Initially, shame about one's faults and weaknesses was fairly common. To be seen and accepted in the group allow the men to get a new perspective, one that goes beyond the self-limiting view each had privately held prior. The value of the safe but honest space of the group can be acknowledged. Carlton's fears about not being able to carry over his momentum without the group suggest that he has allowed himself to feel some of the dependency conflict most men try to avoid. The other conflict zones have also been encountered. Michael's desire to be more masculine and Tony's response that it is fine for him to be who he is address the idealized masculine self-structures with which most men struggle. At this stage, the men are also more comfortable with the idea of "being" with their emotional selves rather than trying to always take action. The group acts as a container of the emotion. The container permits the members to spend some time on the feeling level without having to fix the problems immediately. By more fully embracing the depth of the issue, solutions tend to be more holistic and less like Band-Aids.

Each man's portal to depth has been found over the course of the group. The painful wounds explored in the company of trusted companions are healing.

## Practical Tips

- Because there is a tendency to deny endings, it is important for the group leader to keep this reality in the foreground. Typically, the reminder stirs up feelings of loss and a desire to hold on by members.
- In a final group, structured exercises that encourage the giving and receiving of feedback are paramount. Consolidating learning and discussing how it might be applied in the outside world is a way to keep the group experience alive in each individual.
- In the earliest stage of group, it is important for the members to articulate their goals, knowing that these may shift as the process unfolds. It might be appropriate to revisit these goals at the end of the group sessions to help the men reflect on their progress.
- I like a combination of formal group and an informal potluck in the final session. This manifests the reality of the group ending, celebrates the group's accomplishments in the realm of intimacy, and reminds members that they can take their learning to their individual lives.

# 13

# Starting a Deepening Psychotherapy Group in Your Practice

> What kept coming to mind last evening was that denial of self, of truth, or of our history, is a cancer on the spirit, a fungus on the soul . . . a guy walking with an unnecessary leg cast. There was reference last night to the fear of being judged. Most of the time, the only fair, rational judgment is we are innocent, or we were innocent, or at the very most clueless, and so how can we validate punishing ourselves if we are not guilty of anything but being human, being male?
>
> —Men's group member

There is a need for therapeutic men's groups. There are not enough of them. Men come from a 100-mile radius to attend our group. I believe that if you had the interest to get a group going, you would find that therapists in your area would make referrals to it. As documented in this book, many men who have taken the step to go to individual therapy benefit from the interactions with other men who are focused on self-improvement and interpersonal growth. In this chapter I focus on some practical questions you, as a practitioner, may be wondering about in this regard.

## HOW DO YOU DECIDE ON THE FOCUS FOR YOUR MEN'S GROUP?

Although men have been gathering in groups for most of history, the concept of an intentional psychologically based men's group is relatively new. The Veterans Administration (VA) has used men's groups as a core part of their treatment for war trauma. After the AIDS crisis in the 1980s, men's groups

http://dx.doi.org/10.1037/0000132-014
*Deepening Group Psychotherapy With Men: Stories and Insights for the Journey,*
by F. E. Rabinowitz

supported men dying of the disease, as well as their partners and caregivers. In the early 1990s, Robert Bly led a movement for men reclaiming their more traditional masculine strength. These groups involved storytelling, rituals, and weekend retreats to help men re-own lost male qualities of strength and bravery and balance the era's perceived feminization of masculinity. In more recent years, the ManKind Project has standardized mythopoetic retreats for men (Kauth, 2015).

The therapeutic men's group evolved from 1970s consciousness raising and from the women's and human potential movements. These groups encouraged participants to challenge their gender role conditioning in order to make choices about how to best live in society. Therapeutic men's groups have embraced the findings from the new psychology of men, which has questioned traditional male gender roles, and supported the expansion of the male "toolbox" to enhance emotional, interpersonal, and psychological functioning (Andronico, 1999). The group I lead in Redlands has evolved into a community support structure that allows men from different walks of life to have a place to let down and work on issues, where feedback and authenticity are valued. Although new members are oriented by the leader, returning members informally reinforce the group values, boundaries, and relational connections in early sessions.

Many men's groups focus on specific behaviors and/or situations in which men may find themselves. Men's groups have been conducted with teenage boys (Kiselica, 2005), expectant fathers (Levant, 1996), recently divorced and separated men (Buser & Sternes, 2008; Nahon & Lander, 2008), men with substance abuse problems (Calamari, Cox, & Roth, 1996), domestic violence and anger management (Babcock, Green, & Robie, 2004; Caplan & Thomas, 1995), prison incarceration and release (Lazur, 1996), childhood abuse (Gartner, 1997; Sharpe, Selley, Low, & Hall, 2001), posttraumatic stress in military veterans (Shields, Kuhl, & Westwood, 2017), depression (Rabinowitz, 2005; Rabinowitz & Cochran, 2008), unemployment (Murphey & Shillingford, 2012), and personal growth (Rabinowitz, 2014a, 2014b). By using the principles of building trust, enhancing interpersonal skills, promoting self-awareness, and learning emotional self-control, these groups have been effective in helping men with specific concerns.

## WHERE DO YOU FIND POTENTIAL GROUP MEMBERS, AND WHAT IS THE PROCESS FOR SCREENING AND INTERVIEWING?

There are built-in male populations in certain settings, such as the VA hospital inpatient or outpatient units. Correctional facilities, drug and alcohol rehabilitation programs, community mental health clinics, and psychiatric hospitals also may have ready-made potential male participants. In the general community setting of the nonidentified psychiatric population, it may be more difficult to find male clients ready to volunteer for a men's group.

I have found that groups that are advertised online through therapy practice websites offer a man a private way of finding assistance (e.g., https://www.psychologytoday.com, https://www.goodtherapy.org). By highlighting "men's issues" as the primary focus of your practice, men who are surfing the web can make inquiries to you personally and allow for contact that might not have occurred because of the potential shame about asking for help. Other clinicians in your area may also be made aware of your group through targeted e-mail and social media. Many men in our group have been referred from clinicians who see a men's group as a next step or adjunct to individual work.

Once a man has contacted me by either phone or e-mail, I invite him in for an in-person interview. The interview is to ensure that the group is mutually a good fit and to rule out severe pathology that might hinder the other group members from benefitting. I usually give a general history of our group, its purpose, and the types of issues we talk about in our sessions. Screening question examples include the following: Can you tell me about your own personal story and how being in a men's group seems like a good avenue for you right now? What makes you look forward to an experience like this, and what makes you hesitant? What is your previous experience with counseling and therapy? What worked or didn't work for you in that modality?

A man is going to feel anxious in this type of meeting, so it is important to reframe it as a "getting to know you" interaction. I commend any man who makes it in to see me on this act of strength and desire to live a better life.

## WHAT KIND OF PROBLEMS CAN ARISE WHEN MEN ARE MANDATED TO COME TO A MEN'S GROUP?

Many men are unlikely to voluntarily attend a group unless they have been heavily encouraged or mandated because of legal problems or because of offensive behavior or they have been heavily encouraged by employers or family members. Men who are not intrinsically motivated to change present potential problems in that they are likely to need some time to get used to the expectation of openness and honesty in group interaction. Some may not have ever been in this type of environment. If the whole group is made up of individuals who have been mandated or referred in this way, the group structure should be modeled to take this into account. For instance, an anger management or domestic violence men's group might have a structured curriculum that reinforces the ideas of personal responsibility for actions while still encouraging an openness to self-exploration (see Wexler, 2013). If a man who has been mandated comes to a voluntary group, he should be screened for openness to the experience. In the interview, this individual needs to be introduced to the goals, ideals, and behaviors expected in the group setting. Members who feel coerced by outside forces might need to be reminded of their commitment to openness and authenticity as well as encouraged to acknowledge to the group when sharing is painful or difficult.

## WHAT ARE THE POTENTIAL ISSUES WITH MOVING MALE CLIENTS FROM INDIVIDUAL TO GROUP PSYCHOTHERAPY?

As depicted in previous chapters, the men in the group were first introduced to the therapeutic process by being in individual counseling. The one-on-one nature of psychotherapy allowed each man an individual response for a tailoring of the encounter based on the individual's personality structure, interpersonal style, and background. The group environment is very different. Each man must "compete" for airtime and will not get the same individual attention. The benefit, however, is the interaction, feedback, and support that come from getting to know others who are also engaged in personal growth and healing. It would be important to assess whether your client would be served by an interactive group experience and connection with other men as a part of his learning process. I have included a section at the end of each chapter on individual therapy that highlights the reasons I thought this particular man would benefit from the group. I have also found it important to let him know that he is still welcome to have individual sessions as needed. This allays the fear of abandonment, especially if the individual is going to a group that is not being led by the individual therapist.

## WHAT ARE THE BENEFITS OF COLEADING A MEN'S GROUP?

For most of the time I have led groups, I have had a coleader. As mentioned in Chapter 3, a coleader is able to be another set of eyes on what is occurring with individuals and the group dynamic as a whole. Often, a cofacilitator can observe how other participants are reacting while the other clinician focuses in on an individual or a specific conversation. It is advantageous to have a colleague with whom to discuss the group before and after sessions. Insights about individual reactions, group dynamics, and potential problems are more easily identified with two leaders.

## WHAT ABOUT A FEMALE COLEADER?

In certain settings like the VA, it is not unusual to have a male–female leadership team facilitating a men's therapy group. This configuration often changes the dynamics of the group initially but does not necessarily make the group any less effective. Although some men may find talking about sex, anger, or shame in front of a female clinician difficult at first, the way the female clinician responds can impact how open men are in sharing. As mentioned in Chapter 4, if a female leader demonstrates a nonjudgmental, nonreactive acceptance of whatever men discuss, she will likely earn the male participants' trust over time. It may be very effective for men to confront their issues about women by talking about what they might be holding back in the group because of the female presence. The downside of having a female leader in a men's group is, in my observation, that men in social situations tend to defer to women to monitor and facilitate interpersonal discourse. This could result in some abrogation of responsibility by group members for initiating interpersonal contact and relying on the woman in an authority position to regulate the interactions. In addition, there is some evidence to suggest that men may be motivated to compete for the woman's attention in this kind of situation, leading to a familiar socialized dynamic. Obviously, if these dynamics are occurring, they can be identified by the leaders and used as springboards for reflection and growth within the group.

## WHAT ARE THE ETHICAL ISSUES YOU SEE IN A MEN'S GROUP AROUND RELATIONSHIPS AND BOUNDARIES?

Because many men who attend therapeutic men's groups are seeking interpersonal connection, boundary situations arise. As the leader of the group, I abide by the confidentiality of our communication. This is not necessarily a standard for the members. I have participants sign informed consents about confidentiality and the times when danger to self or others would make it appropriate for me to break this confidentiality. Even although members are encouraged not to break confidentiality, inadvertent breaches can impact trust levels. The most likely occurrence would be when members meet outside of the designated group time and talk with one another. They may meet in settings that are public and use individual names without regard for how others in the environment might interpret their discussion. It is a good idea to talk about confidentiality both in the screening interview and again in early part of the group. If a situation does arise, it is certainly appropriate to bring it up again and talk about the benefits of confidentiality as a precursor to interpersonal trust. Other potential breaches can occur with electronic communication. Our group has a private e-mail list, and the men can interact with one another virtually between group sessions. It is an unlikely but slight possibility that someone not in the group (a partner, relative, friend) could access this conversation and break the confidentiality of the group in this manner.

Subgrouping is the other dynamic that can cause a rift in the group and lead certain members to feel as if they are not being included. Subgrouping occurs when individuals from the group meet or talk with one another outside the official group time. Although this is hard to prevent, the best intervention is to encourage the men to bring outside discussions into the group meeting so that others are aware of these contacts. It is not unusual for some of the men, who share their intimate lives, to become close to other members. Without malice, they may engage in activities outside the group that exclude regular attending members. Again, it is incumbent upon the leader to encourage members to make these interactions public so that others, who may not have the time or resources to participate, know that these other relationships are occurring. The transparency of this approach tends to maintain trust, even when not all can participate in out-of-group activities.

## WHAT SEEM TO BE THE BEST TYPES OF INTERVENTIONS IN A MEN'S GROUP?

Although one could write a book on nothing but interventions in the group situation, the reality is that a clinician should be well versed in a variety of modalities as well as an understanding of group process. A sampling of the best sources to learn more about group therapy process includes G. Corey (2016); M. S. Corey, Corey, and Corey (2010); Kottler and Englar-Carlson (2014); and Yalom (2005).

The interventions used in a men's group will vary based on the focus of the group and the leader's strengths as a clinician. I have identified sample interventions founded on the conflict zones in Chapter 4. In addition to the conflict zones, certain exercises might best be used based on the stage of the group and the receptivity of the group to experiment. The dynamics of a group of men meeting to work on themselves often bring the issues of trust, power, manhood, competition, and vulnerability into discussions without much prompting. At other times, it is important for the leader to have some structured exercises to employ, especially if the group is in a period of resistance or ambivalence about direction. Most of the interventions I use deepen the conversations between members, encouraging exploration of issues that are accompanied by strong emotion and integrating intellectual understanding and body awareness.

Psychodynamic interventions include connecting current experience to childhood issues, interpreting dreams that are brought in by group members, and suggesting that individuals account for the unconscious motivation of their actions inside and outside of the group. Person-centered interventions include active listening before responding to another member's sharing and practicing empathy for others' experiences and emotional sharing. Gestalt interventions include empty-chair conversations with significant individuals in one's life; psychodrama reenactments with group members playing parts in a man's dynamics; and the encouragement of individuals taking responsibility for their projections, reactions, and judgments of another man's sharing. Interpersonal interventions include using the interactions in the here and now of the group to help individuals understand the way they communicate and the emotional impact they have on fellow members. This kind of learning transfers well to relationships outside the group.

Existential interventions focus mainly on highlighting choices, conceptualizing each man as being on a unique but universal journey, and encouraging the search for meaning in one's actions and dreams. Body-oriented interventions include promoting guided meditation and imagery, using a punching bag for anger release, and making use of group members holding another participant as both support and a way to manifest a physical experience of one's own psychological resistance.

## WHAT DO MEN'S GROUP PARTICIPANTS SAY IS HELPFUL FOR THEM?

To answer this question, I present a summary of qualitative survey data of recent men's group members. Members from my group over the past 3 years were solicited to respond anonymously to the following questions. Although there is built-in bias and no control group, the findings do give the reader a sense of how the men frame their experience in the group when asked to reflect. The aggregate responses of 15 individuals have been grouped thematically. These responses might be relevant for your use in the marketing of a men's group in your community.

### What Do You Most Appreciate About Participating in the Men's Group?

- Regularity of meetings and contact with the other members
- Receiving feedback from others
- Unconditional support, acceptance, and concern
- Sense of camaraderie with others who value self-awareness and personal growth
- Safe place to express vulnerable emotions like sadness, loss, fear, anxiety, anger
- A place to experiment with new behavior in response to life stressors
- Learning skills to navigate personal, professional, relational, existential challenges
- Learning to listen better
- Interventions and challenges that push me out of my comfort zone of my usual coping methods
- Hearing multiple perspectives on common themes that men face
- Value hearing other men's stories and struggles

### What Are the Most Difficult Elements for You in the Group?

- Trusting others with personal issues
- Exposing shame and personal weaknesses
- Self-doubt that comes after sharing
- Not always getting the level of support anticipated
- Wanting to rationally problem solve others' issues rather than letting them discover solutions on their own
- Hearing diverse points of views can be uncomfortable
- Relationships with group members when not in the group sessions

- Staying fully present when others are speaking
- Differences in expression of introverts and extroverts
- Dealing with conflict between group members
- Confronting group dynamics when uncomfortable
- Too much intellectualization at times
- Not making enough progress on recurring therapeutic issues

### How Do You Handle the Conflict Between What Is Expected of You as a Man in Society and Being Authentic and Genuine With Yourself and Others?

- Tendency to hide behind male normative behaviors in public settings
- Tendency to put my authentic self on the back burner to gain acceptance and love
- Avoid situations and environments where authenticity is not valued
- Compartmentalize my more sensitive side in nonintimate situations
- Learn to not to care as much about how I am being perceived by others

### What Tangible Benefits Has Group Participation Provided You?

- Learned to trust men again
- Higher level of self-confidence
- Better communication and boundaries in relationships
- Feel more comfortable with being intimately connected in relationships
- Less use of isolation as a way to cope with difficult emotions
- Not as judgmental and self-condemning
- Less likely to be depressed
- Less likely to engage in destructive habits
- Better understanding of childhood influences on current behavior

## FINAL THOUGHTS

It is clear to me that in a world that values strength, bravery, and sacrifice, men are expected to embody these qualities every day of their lives. This pressure affects most men but is rarely acknowledged. When it is difficult to maintain the facade of strength, many men will hide, retreat, or disappear—if not physically, then emotionally. They look around at the outside personas of others and compare them with their more deeply felt insides and feel shame about who they are. The shame is fueled by a sense that they are not living up to the ideals around them, unaware that this process is being experienced by most of the men around them. Those few men who make their way to a therapist may find relief in being able to talk about what they are going through. The men who come to a men's group are able to witness other men from the inside and realize that they are not alone in their struggles.

As articulated by several men in the group, the safe setting provides a forum for being genuine about what one is really feeling and thinking.

Although not an easy process, taking risks to share the inner world and letting oneself be impacted by others feels relieving. Men in the group have an outlet to share their frustration, anger, grief, and fear while getting supportive feedback to carry on with their life journeys. Depression seems to be more of a coping mechanism to tamp down these emotions into a dull, numbing, dark container. The group encourages these inner expressions to be voiced and, in the process, breaks the logjam of depressive thinking and mood. Anxiety, excitement, and passion can emerge as a response to seeing, feeling, and acknowledging one's depth.

It is an uphill battle to counter the cultural forces that value only strength and stoicism in the face of difficult life circumstances. The collective effort of the group is a powerful motivator to change the narrative. One man's willingness to share his struggle is like a domino in pushing another man to take the risk himself. This group dynamic allows men to be both courageous and brave in their authentic sharing of their experience, as well as helpful and therapeutic with their support of their fellow members. The result of the process is often an emotionally freed-up man, with multiple coping mechanisms and increased interpersonal sensitivity, capable of both inner and outer bravery.

# REFERENCES


Addis, M. E. (2011). *Invisible men: Men's inner lives and the consequences of silence.* New York, NY: Times Books.

Addis, M. E., & Hoffman, E. (2017). Men's depression and help-seeking through the lenses of gender. In R. F. Levant & Y. J. Wong (Eds.), *The psychology of men and masculinities* (pp. 171–196). Washington, DC: American Psychological Association.

Addis, M. E., & Mahalik, J. R. (2003). Men, masculinity, and the contexts of help seeking. *American Psychologist, 58,* 5–14. http://dx.doi.org/10.1037/0003-066X.58.1.5

Ainsworth, M. D. (1969). Object relations, dependency, and attachment: A theoretical review of the infant–mother relationship. *Child Development, 40,* 969–1025. http://dx.doi.org/10.2307/1127008

American Psychological Association. (2015). Guidelines for psychological practice with transgender and gender nonconforming people. *American Psychologist, 70,* 832–864. Retrieved from https://www.apa.org/practice/guidelines/transgender.pdf

Andronico, M. P. (Ed.). (1999). *Men in groups: Insights, interventions, and psychoeducational work.* Washington, DC: American Psychological Association.

Babcock, J. C., Green, C. E., & Robie, C. (2004). Does batterers' treatment work? A meta-analytic review of domestic violence treatment. *Clinical Psychology Review, 23,* 1023–1053. http://dx.doi.org/10.1016/j.cpr.2002.07.001

Barry, D., Kovaleski, S., Robertson, C., & Alvarez, L. (2012, April 1). Race, tragedy, and outrage collide after a shot in Florida. *The New York Times.* Retrieved from https://www.nytimes.com/2012/04/02/us/trayvon-martin-shooting-prompts-a-review-of-ideals.html

Bly, R. (1990). *Iron John: A book about men.* New York, NY: Addison-Wesley.

Bowlby, J. (1988). *A secure base.* New York, NY: Basic Books.

Bromet, E., Andrade, L. H., Hwang, I., Sampson, N. A., Alonso, J., de Girolamo, G., . . . Kessler, R. C. (2011). Cross-national epidemiology of *DSM–IV* major depressive episode. *BMC Medicine, 9,* 90. http://dx.doi.org/10.1186/1741-7015-9-90

Brooks, G. R. (1996). Treatment for therapy resistant men. In M. P. Andronico (Ed.), *Men in groups* (pp. 7–20). Washington, DC: American Psychological Association.

Brooks, G. R. (1998a). Group therapy for traditional men. In W. Pollack & R. Levant (Eds.), *New psychotherapy for men* (pp. 83–96). New York, NY: Wiley.

Brooks, G. R. (1998b). *A new psychotherapy for traditional men.* San Francisco, CA: Jossey-Bass.

Brooks, G. R. (2010). *Beyond the crisis of masculinity: A transtheoretical model for male-friendly therapy.* Washington, DC: American Psychological Association. http://dx.doi.org/10.1037/12073-000

Brooks, G. R. (2017). Counseling, psychotherapy, and psychosocial interventions for boys and men. In R. F. Levant & Y. J. Wong (Eds.), *The psychology of men and masculinities* (pp. 317–345). Washington, DC: American Psychological Association.

Brower, V. (2006). Mind–body research moves towards the mainstream. *EMBO Reports, 7,* 358–361. http://dx.doi.org/10.1038/sj.embor.7400671

Burlingame, G. M., MacKenzie, K. R., & Straus, B. (2004). Small-group treatment: Evidence for effectiveness and mechanisms of change. In M. J. Lambert (Ed.), *Bergin and Garfield's handbook of psychotherapy and behavior change* (5th ed., pp. 647–696). New York, NY: Wiley.

Buser, S. J., & Sternes, G. F. (2008). *The guys' guide to getting over divorce.* Houston, TX: Bayou.

Calamari, J. E., Cox, W. M., & Roth, J. D. (1996). Group treatment for men with alcohol problems. In M. Andronico (Ed.), *Men in groups* (pp. 305–322). Washington, DC: American Psychological Association.

Caldwell, L. D., & White, J. L. (2005). African-centered therapeutic and counseling interventions for African American males. In G. Brooks & G. Good (Eds.), *The new handbook of psychotherapy and counseling with men* (pp. 737–753). San Francisco, CA: Jossey-Bass.

Caplan, T., & Thomas, H. (1995). Safety and comfort, content and process: Facilitating open group work for men who batter. *Social Work with Groups, 18,* 33–51. http://dx.doi.org/10.1300/J009v18n02_04

Centers for Disease Control and Prevention. (2015). *National suicide statistics at a glance.* Retrieved from https://www.cdc.gov/violenceprevention/pdf/suicide-datasheet-a.pdf

Chan, R. K., & Hayashi, K. (2010). Gender roles and help-seeking behavior: Promoting professional help among Japanese men. *Journal of Social Work, 10,* 243–262. http://dx.doi.org/10.1177/1468017310369274

Chodorow, N. (1978). *The reproduction of mothering.* Berkeley: University of California Press.

Cochran, S. V. (2005). Assessing and treating depression in men. In G. Brooks & G. Good (Eds.), *The new handbook of psychotherapy and counseling with men* (pp. 229–245). San Francisco, CA: Jossey-Bass.

Cochran, S. V., & Rabinowitz, F. E. (1996). Men, loss and psychotherapy. *Psychotherapy: Theory, Research, Practice, Training, 33,* 593–600. http://dx.doi.org/10.1037/0033-3204.33.4.593

Cochran, S. V., & Rabinowitz, F. E. (2000). *Men and depression: Clinical and empirical perspectives*. San Diego, CA: Academic Press.

Cohn, A. M., & Zeichner, A. (2006). Effects of masculine identity and gender role stress on aggression in men. *Psychology of Men & Masculinity, 7*, 179–190. http://dx.doi.org/10.1037/1524-9220.7.4.179

Connors, J., & Caple, R. (2005). A review of group systems theory. *Journal for Specialists in Group Work, 30*, 93–110. http://dx.doi.org/10.1080/01933920590925940

Corey, G. (2016). *Theory and practice of group counseling* (9th ed.). Boston, MA: Cengage.

Corey, M. S., Corey, G., & Corey, C. (2010). *Groups: Process and practice* (8th ed.). Belmont, CA: Brooks/Cole.

Courtenay, W. (2011). *Dying to be men: Psychosocial, environmental, and biobehavioral directions in promoting health of men and boys*. New York, NY: Routledge. http://dx.doi.org/10.4324/9780203853245

David, D. S., & Brannon, R. (Eds.). (1976). *The forty-nine percent majority: The male sex role*. Reading, MA: Addison-Wesley.

Day, S. X. (2007). *Groups in practice*. Boston, MA: Houghton Mifflin.

Englar-Carlson, M., Evans, M., & Duffey, T. (Eds.). (2014). *A counselor's guide to working with men*. Alexandria, VA: American Counseling Association.

Englar-Carlson, M., & Kiselica, M. S. (2013). Affirming the strengths of men: A positive masculinity approach to assisting male clients. *Journal of Counseling & Development, 91*, 399–409. http://dx.doi.org/10.1002/j.1556-6676.2013.00111.x

Englar-Carlson, M., & Stevens, M. A. (Eds.). (2006). *In the room with men: A casebook of therapeutic change*. Washington, DC: American Psychological Association. http://dx.doi.org/10.1037/11411-000

Englar-Carlson, M., & Stevens, M. A. (2014). Creating experiential weekend retreats for men. In A. B. Rochlen & F. E. Rabinowitz (Eds.), *Breaking barriers in counseling men: Insights and innovations* (pp. 88–98). New York, NY: Routledge.

Farrell, W. (1975). *The liberated man*. New York, NY: Random House.

Fasteau, M. (1974). *The male machine*. New York, NY: McGraw-Hill.

Fenell, D. L. (2014). Counseling stoic warriors: Providing therapy to military men. In M. Englar-Carlson, M. Evans, & T. Duffey (Eds.), *A counselor's guide to working with men* (pp. 227–246). Alexandria, VA: American Counseling Association.

Franklin, A. J. (1998). Treating anger in African American men. In W. S. Pollack & R. F. Levant (Eds.), *New psychotherapy for men* (pp. 239–258). New York, NY: Wiley.

Freud, S. (1910). The origin and development of psychoanalysis. *The American Journal of Psychology, 21*, 181–218. http://dx.doi.org/10.2307/1413001

Gartner, R. B. (1997). An analytic group for sexually abused men. *International Journal of Group Psychotherapy, 47*, 373–383. http://dx.doi.org/10.1080/00207284.1997.11490835

Gilmore, D. D. (1991). *Manhood in the making: Cultural concepts of masculinity*. New Haven, CT: Yale University Press.

Gjerde, F., Block, J., & Block, J. H. (1988). Depressive symptoms and personality during late adolescence: Gender differences in the externalization–internalization of symptom expression. *Journal of Abnormal Psychology, 97*, 475–486. http://dx.doi.org/10.1037/0021-843X.97.4.475

Goldberg, H. (1976). *The hazards of being male*. New York, NY: Nash.

Good, G. E., Dell, D. M., & Mintz, L. B. (1989). Male role and gender role conflict: Relationships to help seeking in men. *Journal of Counseling Psychology, 36*, 295–300. http://dx.doi.org/10.1037/0022-0167.36.3.295

Gough, B., & Robertson, S. (2017). A review of research on men's physical health. In R. F. Levant & Y. J. Wong (Eds.), *The psychology of men and masculinities* (pp. 197–228). Washington, DC: American Psychological Association.

Henretty, J. R., & Levitt, H. M. (2010). The role of therapist self-disclosure in psychotherapy: A qualitative review. *Clinical Psychology Review, 30*, 63–77. http://dx.doi.org/10.1016/j.cpr.2009.09.004

Jung, C. G. (1983). *The essential Jung*. Princeton, NJ: Princeton University Press.

Kaufman, G. (1992). *Shame: The power of caring*. Rochester, VT: Schenkman Books.

Kauth, B. (2015). *A circle of men: The original manual for men's support groups* (2nd ed.). London, England: Silverlight.

Keen, S. (1992). *Fire in the belly: On being a man*. New York, NY: Bantam Books.

Kessler, R. C., Berglund, P., Demler, O., Jin, R., Koretz, D., Merikangas, K. R., . . . National Comorbidity Survey Replication. (2003). The epidemiology of major depressive disorder: Results from the National Comorbidity Survey Replication (NCS-R). *Journal of the American Medical Association, 289*, 3095–3105. http://dx.doi.org/10.1001/jama.289.23.3095

Kilmartin, C., & Smiler, A. P. (2015). *The masculine self*. Cornwall-on-Hudson, NY: Sloan.

Kimmel, M. S. (2017). *Manhood in America: A cultural history* (4th ed.). New York, NY: Oxford University Press.

Kiselica, M. S. (2005). A male-friendly therapeutic process with school-age boys. In G. R. Brooks & G. E. Good (Eds.), *The new handbook of psychotherapy and counseling with men* (pp. 43–58). San Francisco, CA: Jossey Bass.

Kohut, H. (1977). *The restoration of the self*. New York, NY: International Universities Press.

Kottler, J. A., & Englar-Carlson, M. (2014). *Learning group leadership: An experiential approach* (3rd ed.). Thousand Oaks, CA: Sage.

Lazur, R. F. (1996). Managing boundaries: Group therapy with incarcerated adult male sexual offenders. In M. Andronico (Ed.), *Men in groups* (pp. 389–410). Washington, DC: American Psychological Association.

Levant, R. F. (1996). The male code and parenting: A psychoeducational approach. In M. Andronico (Ed.), *Men in groups* (pp. 229–242). Washington, DC: American Psychological Association.

Levant, R. F. (1998). Desperately seeking language: Understanding, assessing, and treating normative male alexithymia. In W. S. Pollack & R. F. Levant (Eds.), *New psychotherapy for men* (pp. 35–56). New York, NY: Wiley.

Levant, R. F., & Powell, W. A. (2017). The gender role strain paradigm. In R. F. Levant & Y. J. Wong (Eds.), *The psychology of men and masculinities* (pp. 15–43). Washington, DC: American Psychological Association. http://dx.doi.org/10.1037/0000023-002

Levit, D. B. (1991). Gender differences in ego defenses in adolescence: Sex roles as one way to understand the differences. *Journal of Personality and Social Psychology, 61*, 992–999. http://dx.doi.org/10.1037/0022-3514.61.6.992

Mahalik, J. R., Locke, B. D., Theodore, H., Cournoyer, R. J., & Lloyd, B. F. (2001). A cross-national and cross-sectional comparison on men's gender role conflict and its relationship to social intimacy and self-esteem. *Sex Roles, 45*, 1–14. http://dx.doi.org/10.1023/A:1013008800019

Mahler, M., Pine, F., & Bergman, A. (1975). *The psychological birth of the human infant*. New York, NY: Basic Books.

Majors, R., & Gordon, J. U. (Eds.). (1994). *The American Black male: His present status and future*. Chicago, IL: Nelson-Hall.

McKelley, R. A. (2014). Pushing haystacks and cracking steel balls: Using metaphors with men. In A. B. Rochlen & F. E. Rabinowitz (Eds.), *Breaking barriers in counseling men: Insights and innovations* (pp. 9–19). New York, NY: Routledge.

Monk, D., & Ricciardelli, L. A. (2003). Three dimensions of the male gender roles as correlates of alcohol and cannabis involvement in your Australian men. *Psychology of Men & Masculinity, 4*, 57–69. http://dx.doi.org/10.1037/1524-9220.4.1.57

Murphey, C. M., & Shillingford, M. A. (2012). Supporting unemployed, middle-aged men: A psychoeducational group approach. *Journal of Employment Counseling, 49*, 85–96. http://dx.doi.org/10.1002/j.2161-1920.2012.00009.x

Nadal, K. L., & Rivera, D. P. (2014). Navigating multiple identities with gay and bisexual men of color. In A. B. Rochlen & F. E. Rabinowitz (Eds.), *Breaking barriers in counseling men* (pp. 156–165). New York, NY: Routledge.

Nahon, D., & Lander, N. R. (2008). Recruitment and engagement in men's psychotherapy groups: An integrity model, value-based perspective. *International Journal of Men's Health, 7*, 218–236. http://dx.doi.org/10.3149/jmh.0703.218

Nolen-Hoeksema, S. (1990). *Sex differences in depression*. Palo Alto, CA: Stanford University Press.

Norcross, J. C., & Lambert, M. J. (2011). Psychotherapy relationships that work II. *Psychotherapy, 48*, 4–8. http://dx.doi.org/10.1037/a0022180

O'Neil, J. M. (Ed.). (2008). Summarizing 25 years of research on men's gender role conflict using the Gender Role Conflict Scale: New research paradigms and clinical implications. *The Counseling Psychologist, 36*, 358–445. http://dx.doi.org/10.1177/0011000008317057

O'Neil, J. M. (2015). *Men's gender role conflict: Psychological costs, consequences, and an agenda for change*. Washington, DC: American Psychological Association. http://dx.doi.org/10.1037/14501-000

Phillips, J. A., Robin, A. V., Nugent, C. N., & Idler, E. L. (2010). Understanding recent changes in suicide rates among the middle-aged: Period or cohort effects? *Public Health Reports, 125*, 680–688. http://dx.doi.org/10.1177/003335491012500510

Pleck, J. H. (1981). *The myth of masculinity*. Cambridge, MA: MIT Press.

Pleck, J. H. (1995). The gender role strain paradigm: An update. In R. F. Levant & W. S. Pollack (Eds.), *A new psychology of men* (pp. 11–32). New York, NY: Basic.

Pollack, W. S. (1995). Deconstructing disidentification: Rethinking psychoanalytic concepts of male development. *Psychoanalytic Psychotherapy, 12*, 30–45.

Pollack, W. S. (1998). Mourning, melancholia, and masculinity: Recognizing and treating depression in men. In W. Pollack & R. Levant (Eds.), *New psychotherapy for men* (pp. 147–166). New York, NY: Wiley.

Pollack, W. S. (1999). *Real boys: Rescuing our sons from the myths of boyhood*. New York, NY: Macmillan.

Pollack, W. S. (2005). "Masked men": New psychoanalytically oriented treatment models for adult and young men. In G. Brooks & G. Good (Eds.), *The new handbook of psychotherapy and counseling with men* (pp. 527–543). San Francisco, CA: Jossey-Bass.

Prochaska, J. O., & Norcross, J. C. (2003). States of change. In J. C. Norcross (Ed.), *Psychotherapy relationships that work: Therapist contributions and responsiveness to patients* (pp. 303–314). New York, NY: Oxford University Press.

Rabinowitz, F. E. (1991). The male-to-male embrace: Breaking the touch taboo in a men's therapy group. *Journal of Counseling & Development, 69,* 574–576. http://dx.doi.org/10.1002/j.1556-6676.1991.tb02648.x

Rabinowitz, F. E. (2005). Group therapy for men. In G. R. Brooks & G. E. Good (Eds.), *The new handbook of psychotherapy and counseling with men* (pp. 603–621). San Francisco, CA: Jossey Bass.

Rabinowitz, F. E. (2006). Thawing the ice man. In M. Englar-Carlson & M. A. Stevens (Eds.), *In the room with men: A casebook of therapeutic change* (pp. 109–127). Washington, DC: American Psychological Association. http://dx.doi.org/10.1037/11411-006

Rabinowitz, F. E. (2014a). Counseling men in groups. In M. Englar-Carlson, M. Evans, & T. Duffey (Eds.), *A counselor's guide to working with men* (pp. 55–70). Alexandria, VA: American Counseling Association.

Rabinowitz, F. E. (2014b). Innovative group counseling with men. In A. B. Rochlen & F. E. Rabinowitz (Eds.), *Breaking barriers in counseling men: Insights and innovations* (pp. 67–76). New York, NY: Routledge.

Rabinowitz, F. E., & Cochran, S. V. (2002). *Deepening psychotherapy with men.* Washington, DC: American Psychological Association. http://dx.doi.org/10.1037/10418-000

Rabinowitz, F. E., & Cochran, S. V. (2008). Men and therapy: A case of masked male depression. *Clinical Case Studies, 7,* 575–591. http://dx.doi.org/10.1177/1534650108319917

Sharpe, J., Selley, C., Low, L., & Hall, Z. (2001). Group analytic therapy for male survivors of childhood sexual abuse. *Group Analysis, 39,* 321–340.

Shepard, D. S. (2002). A negative state of mind: Patterns of depressive symptoms among men with high gender role conflict. *Psychology of Men & Masculinity, 3,* 3–8. http://dx.doi.org/10.1037/1524-9220.3.1.3

Shields, D. M., Kuhl, D., & Westwood, M. J. (2017). Abject masculinity and the military: Articulating a fulcrum of struggle and change. *Psychology of Men & Masculinity, 18,* 215–225. http://dx.doi.org/10.1037/men0000114

Sweet, H. B. (2012). Women working with men: Challenges and opportunities. In H. B. Sweet (Ed.), *Gender in the therapy hour* (pp. 3–18). New York, NY: Routledge. http://dx.doi.org/10.4324/9780203839621

Taub, A. (2017, November 29). How should we respond to sexual harassment? *The New York Times.* Retrieved from https://www.nytimes.com/2017/11/29/upshot/sexual-harassment-response-legal-system-guidelines.html

Trivedi, M. H. (2004). The link between depression and physical symptoms. *Primary Care Companion to the Journal of Clinical Psychiatry, 6*(Suppl. 1), 12–16. Retrieved from https://www.ncbi.nlm.nih.gov/pmc/articles/PMC486942/

U.S. Department of Education, National Center for Education Statistics. (2017). *Status and trends in the education of racial and ethnic groups.* Retrieved from https://nces.ed.gov/fastfacts/display.asp?id=72

Vogel, D. L., Heimerdinger-Edwards, S. R., Hammer, J. H., & Hubbard, A. (2011). "Boys don't cry": Examination of the links between endorsement of masculine norms, self-stigma, and help-seeking attitudes for men from diverse backgrounds. *Journal of Counseling Psychology, 58,* 368–382. http://dx.doi.org/10.1037/a0023688

Wexler, D. B. (2013). *The STOP domestic violence program* (3rd ed.). New York, NY: Norton.

Wexler, D. B. (2014). Approaching the unapproachable: Therapist self-disclosure to de-shame clients. In A. B. Rochlen & F. E. Rabinowitz (Eds.), *Breaking barriers in counseling men* (pp. 30–40). New York, NY: Routledge.

Winnicott, D. (1988). *Human nature*. New York, NY: Schocken Books.

Winter, R. J., & Vallano, J. P. (2016). Black lives matter: Psychological research findings offer ways to foster justice. *Monitor on Psychology, 47*(2), 24.

Wong, Y. J., Liu, T., & Klann, E. M. (2017). The intersection of race, ethnicity, and masculinities: Progress, problems, and prospects. In R. F. Levant & Y. J. Wong (Eds.), *The psychology of men and masculinities* (pp. 262–288). Washington, DC: American Psychological Association.

Yalom, I. D. (1989). *Love's executioner*. New York, NY: Basic Books.

Yalom, I. D. (with Leszcz, M.). (2005). *The theory and practice of group psychotherapy* (5th ed.). New York, NY: Basic Books.

# INDEX

# ABOUT THE AUTHOR

**Fredric E. Rabinowitz, PhD,** is a professor of psychology at the University of Redlands in California. Since 1984, Dr. Rabinowitz has been seeing men in individual, couples, and group psychotherapy in his private practice in Redlands, California. He has coauthored many articles, chapters, and books on counseling men, including *Man Alive: A Primer of Men's Issues* (1995), *Men and Depression* (2000), *Deepening Psychotherapy With Men* (2002), and *Breaking Barriers in Counseling Men* (2014). Dr. Rabinowitz is the past president of the Society for the Psychological Study of Men and Masculinities of the American Psychological Association.